Managing the Health Service

MANAGING
THE HEALTH
SERVICE

S. C. Haywood

Department of Social and Administrative Studies,
Barnett House,
Wellington Square,
Oxford.

WITHDRAWN

London   George Allen & Unwin Ltd
Ruskin House   Museum Street

© George Allen & Unwin Ltd. 1974

ISBN 0 04 350046 3 Hardback
ISBN 0 04 350047 1 Paperback

Printed in Great Britain
by Alden & Mowbray Ltd
at the Alden Press, Oxford

Acknowledgement

I would like to thank all the students on management courses and colleagues whose contributions have sparked off many of the ideas and the form of this book.

Contents

Tables

1
Management in the Health Service

A major theme in the reform of the health service was managerial efficiency.

'. . . it is clear that the creaking structure . . . simply does not match up to modern needs for the delivery of comprehensive health care . . . As the document's brief statement of Government's proposals for a new health service structure makes clear, their essence . . . is the emphasis they place on effective management.'[1]

In the past decade there have been a considerable number of reports on the most appropriate management structure for both the service as a whole[2] and for various personnel operating the services.[3]

A change in the organisational setting in which people work does not in itself solve the problems of the staff responsible for the day-to-day management of the service. The problems of making resources go round; soothing irate staff; co-ordinating the activities of staff who sometimes seem most reluctant to be co-ordinated; coping with the teething troubles of a new project or service; getting the ambulance to the right place at the right time; explaining to the general practitioner why he wasn't told his patient had been discharged or placating the irate patient who has been kept waiting longer than the prescribed thirty minutes after his out-patient appointment time, will still remain.

What this book tries to do is to go beyond – to borrow the Secretary of State's phrase – the 'surfeit of prospectuses' and look at the everyday problems of management. In the end the success of the reform – as the consultative document acknowledged – rests on the 'quality of management'.[4] Or more precisely, perhaps, the calibre of those who manage the service. The focus of this book is these managers and the everyday problems they face.

The theme of the book is the better use of resources. We share

13

the belief of the architects of reform that resources have to be deployed more efficiently and effectively than hitherto. More effective management will free resources at present tied up in inefficient practices and marginally effective services to finance the developments which all want.

In our analysis of the problems of those in the service the perspective employed is not that of the school of the 'principles of management'. We seek rather to deepen understanding of the organisation in which staff work. This approach assumes that a greater appreciation of the way an organisation really works is a prerequisite to better management. Another student of the management of health care has argued that this approach may give 'better returns' in terms of increased effectiveness than courses (or presumably books!) trying to impart 'specific, managerial skills'.[5]

One justification for this approach is the frequently expressed doubts of the general applicability of the 'principles of management'.[6] Our approach to more effective management would, for example, counsel caution on the advantages of a more clearly defined 'line management' in hospitals. Some hospital administrators are more sanguine about its usefulness. Mr A. A. McIver feels in his contribution to *Modern Hospital Management* that many of the administrative difficulties in hospitals would be lessened by the recognition of the administrator as *the* line manager.[7] Perhaps Urwick and Brecht, whom he quotes, would have agreed. Yet other studies of health service agencies and comparable organisations would counsel against such firm expectations. Given the pre-eminent position of the clinical function, the medical profession, the rapid growth in the professions ancillary to medicine, the parallel hierarchies of nurses, administrators and now of doctors, line management of the type Mr McIver has in mind is hardly feasible or perhaps desirable. There will have to be a number of line managements. Our perspective is broader and draws on other theories of management.

An approach of this type requires case material to make it more intelligible (and acceptable) to those who actually run the service. However, case studies in health service management seem sparse. We have therefore drawn primarily on illustrations which come from the author's own experience and were found useful by students on management courses or were produced by the students themselves. Another source on which we draw are the professional journals.

The original subject of the book was hospital management,

which remains the major preoccupation. This is justified on two counts. First, the hospital service will continue to absorb the lion's share of resources. Second, there are more similarities between the management structure of the new service and the hospital service before 1974 (regional authorities, central finance) than with the community services, particularly local health authorities.

We can claim the attention of those in the community service if only because material on hospital management will be of greater information value to them than hitherto. In addition we point to similarities and contrasts, where appropriate, between the management of community and hospital services.

WHO ARE THE MANAGERS?

We have said the book is intended for staff who in some sense are managers. But who are they? There is no easy answer to a question which has vexed, among others, the hospital organisation research unit at Brunel University. As a starting point they regard someone as a manager if he is accountable for the work of his sub-ordinates.[8] If we accept this definition as the group of staff on whose problems we should focus there is an obvious and important omission. It excludes medical staff from the definition of man-ager.[9] It would also exclude heads of departments of a highly professionalised staff who are not directly accountable to him.[10] Medical social workers, biochemists, psychologists, physicists and pharmacists are examples of staff who may fall into this latter category.

Our definition of staff whose needs this book is intended to serve includes these groups. But what precisely is the rationale for including such staff in our definition of managers? One part of the rationale is the important contribution they make to the development of a service. They are not merely instruments of the policy-makers. In the case of social welfare institutions comparable groups of employees were found to 'create and continually modify, the service'.[11]

The other reason for the inclusion of these professional groups in our definition of managers is related to the main theme of the book – the better deployment of existing resources. Many incur expenditure and their decisions play a crucial part in the way resources are used.

Not only is the book addressed to the condition of those who acknowledge themselves to be managers but to other staff, particularly professional and technical, who might be reluctant to see themselves in such a role.

THE PLAN OF THE BOOK

We look first at those features of the health service which many staff see as almost insuperable obstacles to the development of the service. These are the shortage of resources which has beset the service since 1948 and the inadequacy of the organisational structure chosen for it (Chapters 2 to 9). This discussion paves the way for a realistic appraisal of the power of staff in the service (Chapters 10 and 11). The final part of the book concerns itself with the particular contribution they can make to the problems of efficiency (Chapters 12 to 17) and staff/patient relations (Chapters 18 and 19).

2

Shortages

I THE COMMON VIEW

'We are already making £1 do the work of 30/-.' This was the rejoinder of a hospital secretary when the discussion on a management training course turned to the need to improve efficiency in the health service. He was one who felt strongly that the only way to meet the increasing pressures on hospitals in particular was a large infusion of extra resources. This was a prevalent attitude among hospital staff, certainly during the period when Enoch Powell was Minister of Health in the early 1960s. In his subsequent reflections on the hospital service he had some critical things to say about it. 'In every inadequacy the obligation of government to provide is a continuous alibi; one does not have to do something about it oneself if it is the business of the Minister and the Chancellor to put it right.'[1]

Interestingly the attitude has survived both Powell's stewardship and subsequent exposé. Some of the credit for its survival must go to Professor Henry Miller. In a radio discussion with Mr Powell in 1966 he criticised his book in these terms. 'My main criticism would be that you haven't dealt in your book with what I regard as the major problems of medical politics – with our dilapidated plant, our failure to provide staff adequately to man even the existing service, our disproportionate dependence on immigrant doctors and the rising tide of medical emigration.'[2] Not surprisingly the belief that the service has been underfinanced, inadequately staffed and that by implication this was an almost insurmountable obstacle to improvement was voiced at the twentieth anniversary conference of the National Health Service. 'Only if hospitals received more money would a health service be achieved of which all could be proud . . .'[3] was the publicly expressed view of one senior administrator. An even more pessimistic view was expressed by 'Spectator' in a professional journal in the same year. 'Unless the ministry of health and through them the regional hospital boards can hold out some reasonable hope of more money

17

and better facilities in the foreseeable future morale will drop and those who talk about the service being "on the verge of collapse" may well be right.'[4] In 1969 the British Medical Association's planning unit was similarly trenchant on the lack of resources allocated to the health service. 'It is beyond question that overall expenditure on medicine in Britain is below that devoted to it in most other developed countries and far below that necessary for an efficient service. The financial allocation to the health service should be substantially increased.'[5] In the following year *The Hospital*, perhaps with a touch of resignation, reported that 'at the very least it can be said that the service will continue to be hard pressed financially'.[6] Similar views were expressed in the medical press in the same year. 'Certainly until those who organise the health service at the centre set out their long term sums with thought and precision, they must not be surprised if the service attracts less than its due in public monies.'[7] No doubt it was a similar analysis that led the Royal Commission on Medical Education somewhat earlier to recommend a ratio of 1,800 doctors for every million people rather than 1,180 which prevails now.[8]

The views of personnel employed in the health services were shared by others outside the service. Arthur Seldon has long argued that the chronic shortage of resources for all social services has produced a 'crisis' situation.[9] An American academic takes it as an established judgement. 'As we will note later, one of the greatest problems in Great Britain in the past decade – contrary to the usual stereotype – was the failure to invest sufficient funds in health care to fulfil the stated ideals of the British national health service, even in a modest way . . .'[10] Richard Crossman in a public lecture at the University of Hull after leaving office, felt that in the absence of large additional resources for the National Health Service, it was possible to talk about the 'collapse' of the service.[11] He acknowledged that additional resources on a sufficiently large scale to avoid this were unlikely.

This small selection of quotations clearly demonstrates that the convictions about 'inadequate' finance and 'unfair' shares of resources persist into the 1970s. And with this conviction goes the belief, perhaps more clearly demonstrated by the planning committee of the British Medical Association and Professor Miller, that an essential prerequisite for better services is a large increase in resources to the health service. Any book on health service management must therefore start at this point.

Powell found these beliefs and attitudes to be most firmly entrenched in the hospital service. A brief perusal of professional journals indicates that this is probably still so. Powell attributed this to the different methods of financing the community and hospital services. Where there was a more direct link between provision and taxation in the community services, there was a greater realism about the finiteness of resources and less denigration of existing services.[12]

Our examination of the criticisms of under-financing consequently concentrates on the pre-reform hospital service. A further justification is the financial structure of the integrated health service. Like the pre-reform hospital service it will be centrally financed. An examination of the problems of local government financial control would therefore be of historical interest only.

An analysis of these criticisms is an important part in the process of management training. If they are alibis to shift responsibility, as Powell clearly thought they were in the 1960s, then some clarification may open the way for a change in attitude and thus more dynamic management. Or, if it is a legitimate criticism, does it apply to all hospitals and all departments? If not, and overwhelming shortages are localised, should we have different expectations of the ability of various departments, hospitals and areas to meet the increasing demands made of them? If it is not an alibi and the criticisms are justified, it is still necessary to be clear in what sectors there are shortages and in what ways they preclude further substantial gains in efficiency. Only when we are clear about the rights and wrongs of these issues can we reach a considered judgement on the difficulties in developing the service without a substantial increase in resources.

We now turn to a consideration of these issues. In this chapter we look at the financial allocations to the health service and in the next pay particular attention to the share taken by the hospitals. In Chapter 4 we consider the question of staffing in the hospital service and conclude this particular topic in Chapter 5 with a discussion on what does constitute an adequate service, and the implications this has for managers in the integrated health service.

II   HAS THE HEALTH SERVICE BEEN UNDER-FINANCED ?

In recent years the health service has been absorbing a larger share of our national wealth. 1970 was the fifteenth successive year in which the health services increased their share of resources.[13] By 1967 expenditure on the health service accounted for more than 5 per cent of the national income for the first time (see Table 1).

Additional resources have been forthcoming. Health service

Table 1 *Percentage of national income devoted to the National Health Service in selected years since 1948*

Year	NHS Percentage of national income
1950	4·42
1955	3·91
1965	4·62
1967	5·12
1970	5·59

Source: Office of Health Economics information sheets

expenditure in the period of economic difficulties in the late 1960s has grown faster than some pessimists thought possible. All the indications are that this process will continue at about the same rate into the 1970s. In spite of talk about cutting back public expenditure, the revenue allocation to the National Health Service is to be increased more rapidly than the probable increase in national wealth. In one white paper, health and welfare expenditure was expected to rise by 5·1 per cent per annum in real terms between 1971–2 and 1975–6.[14] This compares with a growth of only 2·7 per cent per annum for all public expenditure during the same period. Two members of the Department of Applied Economics at Cambridge have pointed to the similarity between the growth rate planned for the early seventies in the previous white paper and that which was actually achieved between 1960–1 and 1965–6. In the period of 1965–6 and 1970–1 it was one percentage point higher – 4·7 per cent.[15]

An element in the criticisms of public parsimony towards the health service has been a feeling of unfairness: the National Health Service was not getting its due. International comparisons, particularly with the United States, have been utilised to substantiate this criticism. Other countries, it is argued, do spend a higher proportion of their national income on health services than does the United Kingdom.[16] It is surprising how selective these comparisons are. How would health service personnel feel if the British armed forces argued (as no doubt they do) that the United States government spent a higher proportion of their national income on defence and therefore the British services were not getting their fair share of resources? Use of international comparisons to indicate the increasing importance attached to health expenditure as national income rises is also less persuasive now when related to the British situation. The proportion of the national income devoted to the health services is increasing in the United Kingdom too. Another difficulty in using international comparisons to decide the correct allocation to British health services is the difficulty of comparing like with like. Do the higher expenditures elsewhere mean more and better service per patient?

There are those who feel the health services have not received their fair share of resources, but do not base their case on international comparisons: their frame of reference is other public expenditure. The difficulty with this argument is that there is no way of saying what proportion (the same, more or less?) of public expenditure should be allocated to health services. No one would argue too that the proportions should be fixed for all time and each service receive the same percentage increase in resources. And what is the proper balance between expenditure on health, education, housing or welfare services? To argue that health should get a bigger share of available resources is to say that the proportion of unmet need in health was greater than in other social services. Need is too slippery a notion to permit such comparisons, and provide a sound basis for this argument.

In fact the health service in comparison with other social services will do well in the 1970s if the projections of public expenditure made at the beginning of the decade materialise. (See Table 2.)

Table 2 *Acceleration in public spending allowing for the relative price effect*

Programme	Labour Government 1964/5 to 1968/9 actual percentage	First Conservative white paper 1970/1 to 1974/5 planned percentage	Second Conservative white paper 1971/2 to 1975/6 planned percentage
Health	3·9	4·7	5·1
Social security	8·3	2·1	1·5
Education	4·9	4·8	4·5
Aid to industry	9·0	−7·1	−14·4
Defence	−0·7	0·1	1·4
All public expenditure programmes	5·9	2·6	2·7

Source: Rudolph Klein. The *Lancet*, Vol. II for 1971: No. 7737, p. 1307.

In conclusion, it is worth reiterating that in the late 1960s health service expenditure did increase faster than national income.

It is indeed hard to see how accusations of *undue* meanness, unfairness, *gross* under-financing, etc., either in the past or in promised allocations, can be sustained. However, we have identified the hospital sector as the originator of most of the criticisms, so it could be that the hospital service was less generously treated than the other sectors of the health service. We look at the financial resources made available to the hospital service in the next chapter.

3

Have the Hospitals been Under-financed?

I THE SHARE OF THE NHS BUDGET ALLOCATED TO HOSPITALS

The hospitals have been taking a *larger* share of total resources allocated to the health service. In 1965 hospital expenditure took 2·75 per cent of national income; in 1950 it had accounted for only 2·25 per cent.[1] In 1970 the hospital service accounted for 61·8 per cent of total expenditure. This was the highest proportion in the history of the service.[2] It might be argued that this information tells us more about the relative importance attached to the hospital services than it does about the actual resources being made available. How then have hospitals fared in hard cash terms? A larger share of a budget does not in itself indicate adequate consideration has been given to the needs of the service.

In 1970/1 the estimated revenue expenditure on hospitals was £983 million. In 1964/5 it had been £526 million. Allowing for the increase in prices and remuneration this represented an additional investment of £111 million; a real increase in available resources of one fifth.[3] Over a longer period there has been a steady growth in revenue resources allocated to hospitals. And this process will continue. In the White Paper on Public Expenditure to 1975–6 provision is made for current expenditure on the hospital service to increase at constant prices by 4·3 per cent in 1972/3 and 3·5 per cent in subsequent years.[4] What this means in actual financial terms is set out in Table 3.

II THE DISTRIBUTION OF THE INCREMENT

The increment made available to the hospital service varied between 1·71 per cent and 3·36 per cent between 1964/5 and 1970/1 (see Table 4).

A useful way of assessing the relative size of the increment is to relate it to the number of discharged patients. In 1965/6 the

Table 3 *Public expenditure on the health services in the 1970s*

	1970-1 provisional outturn	1971-2 estimate	1972-3 estimate	1973-4 estimate	1974-5 estimate	1975-6 estimate
At 1971 survey prices						
Capital expenditure:						
Hospitals	147·9	174·9	201·5	203·3	204	201
Family practitioner services	0·6	0·3	—	0·7	1	—
Local authority health and personal social services	45·4	58·8	73·6	79·6	81	86
Current expenditure:						
Hospitals	1,215·2	1,266·6	1,320·9	1,366·6	1,415	1,464
Family practitioner services	504·0	495·1	500·3	510·2	523	535
Local authority health and personal social services	326·6	351·0	374·1	405·1	430	460

Source: White Paper on Public Expenditure to 1975/6. HMSO, Cmnd. 4829, 1971.

Table 4   *National Health Service hospital revenue expenditure £ million*

Financial year	Actual expenditure	Increase compared with previous year due to changes in prices and remuneration	Increment	Increment as % of previous year's expenditure
1964/5	526	—	—	—
1965/6	580	45	9	1·71
1966/7	637	42	15	2·59
1967/8	690	35	18	2·83
1968/9	755	48	17	2·46
1969/70	834	55	24	3·18
1970/1*	983	121	28	3·36

* 1970/1 estimated figures
Source: Annual report of the Department of Health and Social Security 1970, p. 291.

increment was just under £2 per head: in 1970/1 it was estimated to be between £5 and £6. Looked at from the point of view of the total budget of a large acute hospital it must seem a minute sum.

However, not all hospitals received an equal share of the improvement monies which were made available. These were, and are more likely both to find their way to particular units or projects (e.g. geriatric and long-stay hospitals in the 1970s) and to hospitals with lower standards. The improvement monies were the only means available to the Department to equalise the standard of hospital services throughout the country. Once budgets for hospitals had been fixed (as they had to be) on what had been spent previously and the option of 'levelling down' rejected, poor hospitals could only be brought nearer the standards of the better ones by giving them a disproportionate share of the improvement monies. Some hospitals or regions with the highest standards in 1948 may have consequently received smaller shares of the improvement monies than our earlier average figures would suggest. Staff employed in those hospitals might have become understandably frustrated.

The process of levelling up will continue into the 1970s as there is still a considerable gap between the expenditure of the richest and poorest regions. Indeed the persistence of the gap raises some doubts about the vigour with which the levelling-up process was in fact pursued in the 1950s and 1960s. Griffiths, in a comparison of current expenditure per head per region from 1955 to 1969/70 has concluded:

'that there are large and persistent inequalities in the levels of expenditure *per capita* on all hospitals. The three worst-off regions, Sheffield, East Anglia and Birmingham remain anchored at the bottom of the league while Oxford and Wessex have drifted downwards away from the average. The extremes between the regions remain as far apart as ever. The top region spent 69 per cent more *per capita* than the bottom region in the early 50s and still spends 64 per cent more *per capita* now . . .'[5]

Even if some of the discontent is explained by the discrimination against the better-off hospitals in the past, it is unlikely to produce a bigger share of the improvement monies in the future. Indeed discrimination could intensify given the avowed intention of the Department to eliminate the disparities in standards over a ten-year period.[6] This suggests that better-off hospitals and regions will see little or even less of the improvement monies allocated to the hospitals in the next ten years, than they perhaps did in the previous decades.

The discontent among the better-off regions cannot, however, be explained by a smaller share of the capital allocation in the past. Bosanquet has argued that the capital programme, at least until 1969, did not in practise seem to equalise standards throughout the country. Looking through the annual report for that year at the location of projects costing more than £1 million he reports: 'of £247 million worth of work in progress involving such schemes, only 29 per cent was being carried out north of the Trent, which had about 39 per cent of the population. Odder still was the high concentration of schemes in the London Area.'[7]

Although one high cost region lies north of the Trent – Liverpool – there is general agreement that facilities in the north are inferior to those farther south. If then the Department in the 1970s couples its increased determination to equalise operational standards with a commitment to give the poorer regions an increasing share of capital resources, then certain hospitals particularly in the South of England are going to see very little of development monies in the next decade.

On top of these factors is the growing determination to upgrade particular services in hospitals. Governments have increasingly emphasised the need for disproportionate development, for example, of geriatric and psychiatric services. The relative neglect

of these services in the last twenty-five years means few would dis-
agree with this objective. However, the rub comes with the limited
amounts of additional resources for 'improvement' (in the last
six years of the previous decade it was less than 4 per cent per
annum). A concentration of improvement monies in particular
services may well reinforce the frustrations of staff in other sectors
of the service.

There is another factor which reduces the visibility and availability of the improvement monies. The budgetary process, if
handled properly, encourages staff to make decisions about priorities and which improvements in service they would most like to
see. They are asked to plan. Yet these plans, based on conscious
decisions, can be pre-empted by other factors; some unexpected,
others anticipated, which serve to reduce choice about priorities
further. For example, demographic changes have pre-empted
resources which could otherwise have been available to allow
a wider range of options. Demographic changes, particularly
the increasing percentage of elderly who make higher demands on
most sectors of the health services, increase expenditure without
improving the quality of existing services. In 1956 Abel Smith
and Titmuss predicted that changes in population structure would
increase expenditure by 8 per cent between 1951 and 1971.[8]
Klein and Ashley point out that costs in the health service have
risen by 60 per cent in real terms over this same period.[9] If the
1956 predictions were accurate then we can say that approximately
one seventh of the additional resources were pre-empted in this
way. More recently, the White Paper on Public Expenditure to
1975/6 estimated that about one quarter of the annual increments
to the hospital service would be required to maintain standards
for the increasing and ageing population.[10] Put more positively,
more than three-quarters of the increased financial allocations
have been available for other improvements and it is not likely
to go below this proportion in the early and mid-1970s.

However, not only demographic factors pre-empt decisions on
the use of improvement monies. Another factor is the rising
expectations of the public, which can lead to an increased demand
for an existing service. The unit at St Thomas' Hospital for
people suffering from permanent respiratory paralysis is a good
example of this process at work. 'The use of respiratory equipment etc. . . . has enabled patients to live nearly normal lives in the
last 3 to 5 years . . . Soon the reputation of the unit spread and
attracted other patients with a similar form of disability to it.'[11]

The net result of the increased demand was a diversion of the hospitals resources, which were said to have remained roughly constant. If resources had been increasing, no doubt some of the increment would have to be diverted to meet this need.

Obviously more effective treatment for a disability clearly constitutes an improvement, as does meeting the greater volume of demand from the elderly. Hypothetically, a clinical decision to meet this type of increased demand may nevertheless pre-empt a previous decision to allocate improvement monies to another needy part of the service. Frustration at seeing improvement monies pre-empted in this way may be exacerbated by the realisation that the diversion of funds is providing more rather than a better quality of service. Where this happens, staff can perhaps be understood when they say the hospitals have been deprived of funds for improvements in service.

This incident also raises the question of the effective control of demand and expenditure. Should increased demand of this type have been met? If so, who should take the decision? In a service in which staff complain so much of shortages, such a decision should be a conscious one in which this course of action is weighed against alternative investments. We shall argue later that an efficient service would try to limit the occasions when expenditure escalates automatically in cases of this type. And to be efficient, a decision to meet increased demand would have to be weighed against the benefits of alternative investments.[12]

Another illustration of a new development almost imperceptibly pre-empting development monies at a national level was provided by Richard Crossman. He said that while he was in office, the sudden use of the drug *L. Dopa* for Parkinsons disease pre-empted £3 million he had earmarked for other purposes.[13] Clearly, the availability of the drug opened up the way for an improved service. Patients could be treated more effectively. The other side of the coin was the possible pre-emption of funds, because of the additional costs, earmarked for improvements in particular sectors of the service. Given the environment in which health service staff have to work, it is clear that there will always be irresistible, sometimes imperceptible, and unexpected claims on the additional resources made available for improvements. Where a situation of this type is accentuated by a below 'average' share of the increment (e.g. as part of the policy of equalising standards), staff may be forgiven if they think improvement monies conspicuous only by their absence. But this is quite a different point to the general criticism about the gross under-financing with which we started.

III HAS THE HOSPITAL SERVICE BEEN UNDER-FINANCED ?

A fuller answer to this question has to wait until we have discussed what adequacy really means in Chapter 5. At this juncture
we can say simply that additional financial resources for the
hospital service (as for the service as a whole) have been forthcoming and at a faster rate than some thought possible. However,
it is still true that *some* have seen and will see very small amounts of
improvement monies. And this small increment could well have
been absorbed by an automatic escalation in demand for the
same service without corresponding improvements in the quality
of service. An important element in the criticism of under-
financing may be the unavailability of improvement monies for
higher standards of service or a reduction of need on a *planned*
basis. Conscious choice may be pre-empted by events or government priorities.

It is in this context that complaints about 'shortage' can be most
sympathetically understood. From the perspective of some,
additional resources with the implications this has for morale and
expectations of better times, must seem negligible. Sympathy,
however, with some, does not substantiate the more generalised
accusations of the unfair treatment of the National Health Service
in general or hospitals in particular. The hospital service in particular has, within a British context, been treated comparatively
generously. For certain hospitals and particular sectors there has
been and will continue to be a real net increase in available funds.
If staff in these hospitals argue that the absence of improvement
monies was and is a major obstacle to improved services, they are
indeed searching for alibis to avoid criticism of their own performance.

4

Is the Health Service Under-staffed?

I FINANCE AND STAFFING

Inability to recruit the number of staff required is not solely explained by the absence of funds. To this extent problems of staffing constitute an independent constraint on improved managerial performance. The absence of suitably qualified technical staff to man renal dialysis units was one such occasion. Kenneth Robinson, then Minister of Health, went to considerable lengths to point out that it was the absence of staff (and other factors) rather than money which was holding up the development of this service.[1] Even given the political will to make funds available on a large scale, it is unlikely that the service can recruit the 10,000 skilled personnel estimated to be required by the planning unit of the British Medical Association.[2] Another obvious example is the recruitment of medical staff. Clearly extra finance would not have an immediate impact on the number of doctors available for at least a decade. To what extent then have shortages of staff been an insuperable obstacle to improvements?

II SHORTAGES: THE COMMON VIEW

Some of the most persistent complaints seem to come from the nurses. For them the word 'shortage' seems as much of a programmed response as the description 'capitalist' in the Russian vocabulary, when referring to someone from the West. As with finance, the 'shortage' of staff, either because they are unavailable or because there are insufficient resources to hire them becomes a convenient byway in any discussion on how services can be improved. It provides all too often a convenient excuse to avoid the (perhaps more painful) examination of the use of existing staff from which the extra resources for development may be found. 'I used frequently to be appalled by the ossification of thought which contemplation of unfilled theoretical "establishments" of nursing staff could induce in otherwise vigorous and go ahead people.'[3]

30

Contemplation of unfilled theoretical establishments, with presumably the same ossification of thought, is a frequent pastime even after this admonition. At the end of 1967 the theatre superintendent told the third annual congress of the national association of theatre nurses that 'many operating theatres are working close to the danger level because of staff shortage and that unless a realistic salary scale is produced . . . operating theatre suites in our new hospitals will become great white elephants'.[4]

Two years later the *Nursing Times* reported that consultants in eleven London teaching hospitals, 'alerted at last to the dangerous shortages of nursing staff in the hospitals . . . have sent the following telegram to Mr Richard Crossman on December 11th . . . Chairmen (of medical advisory committees) feels there is a serious crisis, and urgent solution to the problem essential if standard of our hospital services is to be maintained.'[5] This was in the context of pay negotiations. A year later a leader in the same journal reported 'it is generally believed that there is a shortage of nurses throughout the country', though the writer was more cautious in her judgement of the situation.[6] These are but three examples of a commonly held view by most occupations about themselves. It is not, of course, a phenomenon confined to health service or hospital staff.

III STAFFING: SOME FACTS AND FIGURES

In this section we look mostly at the situation in hospitals since it is from this sector that the most vociferous complaints have come. In the second half of the 1960s, which gave rise to fears of 'crisis and collapse', the number of employed staff in all major hospital occupational groups was increasing (see Table 5). Overall the number of staff available has increased more rapidly than any of the rather simple measures of increased 'demand' we have used. This was true even of nurses who showed the smallest aggregate increase over this period. Since 1949 the total number of hospital nursing staff has risen from 148,812 to over 270,000 in 1970. Similar gains have been made by other grades of staff.

There are three obvious qualifications to this simple comparison of number of staff and demand. First, to what extent is this optimistic picture invalidated by the reduction in the number of hours worked by members of staff? The increase in number of staff employed may have done little more than offset the loss of available manpower through shorter working hours. Second, gains in general do not necessarily mean gains in particular. What about the distribution of the increases within the categories of staff used in the table? This is a particularly important consideration in the case of nurses. Third, the effective demand on hospitals may have increased more than our simple yardsticks suggest. In a given hour staff today may have more demands made on them than their predecessors. The obvious fact that patients, at least on acute wards, are very ill and dependent for a higher proportion of their stay than their predecessors has led to the search for dependency ratios for nurses as a more accurate gauge of their workload.

It is important to assess the importance of these qualifications. First the reduction in the number of hours worked. From our viewpoint the crucial point is whether the number of nursing working hours available, for example, to managers has declined. This was an issue to which the Briggs Committee on Nursing addressed itself. Its conclusion was clear. 'Total nursing and midwifery numbers grew during the 1960s and have reached new heights each year. Even given the reduction in the length of the working week which took place during this period, total working hours available increased.'[7] The committee were talking of nursing resources available to the National Health Service. Both community and hospital services have benefited from the increases.

There is a more positive way of looking at the reduction of the nursing working week than a gloomy analysis of how many pairs of hands are available. The reduction of hours *is* an improvement in itself. To the extent that the reduction is made good by increased recruitment and overtime payments, part of the national increment is being made available to permit a shorter working week. These additional resources could equally have been used for other purposes both outside and within the health service.

Second, there is the question of how the distribution of the increase in numbers has been effected. A large increase in numbers does not mean an equal distribution either geographically or between sectors and grades. In the medical and nursing sector it is the recruitment of midwives, trained nursing staff in psychiatric hospitals and medical staff for accident and emergency services which are thought to present some of the particular difficulties. The Briggs Committee identified a number of 'perceived shortages some of them serious' in nursing. In addition to the obvious ones in geriatric, chronic, long-stay and psychiatric hospitals, they also pointed to the shortages in special units, staff nurses, and in particular parts of the country.[8] They found it

Table 5 *Staffing standards in hospitals, 1966–70, compared with simple indices of workload (England)*

Staff	Numbers 1966	1970	% Increase/decrease
Medical (WTE)	19,094	22,059	15·53
Professional & technical (WTE)	27,603	33,168	20·17
Nurses (WTE)	217,675	237,350	9·04
Maintenance/works domestic full-time	150,122	146,863	−2·18
Part-time	57,886	70,602	21·96

	Numbers 1966	1970	% Increase
Discharges & deaths (000s)	467	5,012	8·56
New outpatient attendances	7,210	7,578	5·10
Total outpatient attendances	29,928	31,844	6·40
Accident & emergency department attendances	12,751	13,322	4·48

Source: Annual Reports of the Ministry of Health and Department of Health and Social Security.

more difficult to pinpoint shortages in the community nursing field.[9]

Even in the field of hospital professional and technical staff where the numbers employed have increased substantially there may still be problem areas. Some observers have pointed out that there was a decrease in the decade 1958 to 1968 in the number of medical social workers, psychiatric social workers and occupational therapists, without any obvious changes in medical practice to explain the decline.[10] In the years 1966–70, however, this was no longer true and the number employed increased (see Table 6).

National aggregates, of course, conceal local difficulties, particularly where total numbers are small. This was forcibly brought home to the author who wanted to include trained social workers in a study involving eleven acute hospitals in the Leeds region. There were insufficient to constitute a meaningful sample. Recruitment of dieticians, trained medical and psychiatric social workers, biochemists and orthoptists, for example, in less favoured areas is no doubt difficult. Briggs also pointed to the difficulties of recruiting nursing staff in certain regions.[11]

We can identify the areas where many of these particular difficulties occur. For example, in the East Anglian Region the proportion of nurses per 1,000 population is 20 per cent below the average for England. The proportion of professional and technical staff per 1,000 population in the Liverpool, Manchester and Sheffield regions is much lower than that for the metropolitan regions.[12] And not all the disparity can be explained by the higher provision of hospital beds in some regions. Bosanquet has pointed to the likelihood of more staff being attracted to the more glamorous areas in the South, particularly London, because of the concentration of new building projects there. Trends in recruitment may continue to make staff less available to certain areas of the country. The attraction, he feels, 'will tend to be at the expense of the older hospitals; and unless there is strong control from the central department, of the country north of the Trent'.[13] In the north, then, non-availability of staff independent of financial constraints may be more of a problem than in the south. Managers in some areas may have more justification when they cite staff shortages as a major justification for the lack of progress. The third qualification to an optimistic view of staffing levels was the changing nature of the work. There are two ways in which the nature of the work may have become more demanding. First, there is more work per patient arising from such factors as shortened length of stay in hospital and more diagnostic and treatment aids per

Table 6 *Number of staff employed in selected occupations in hospitals (England)*

Class of Staff	Whole time equivalents of staff employed		% Increase
	30 September 1966	30 September 1969	
Dietitians	231	281	2·1
Medical laboratory technicians: qualified	3,097	3,556	14·8
Medical Laboratory technicians: students and juniors	4,534	4,884	7·7
Occupational therapists	1,356	1,486	9·6
Physiotherapists	4,229	4,249	0·4
Radiographers: diagnostic	3,651	3,763	3·0
Medical social workers: qualified	773	833	7·7
Psychiatric social workers: qualified	231	263	13·8
Social workers: others with qualifications	162	256	58·0
All classes: total	2,9219	31,430	7·5

Sources: Annual Report of the Ministry of Health 1966.
Annual Report of the Department of Health and Social Security 1969.

patient. Second, the emotional demands on each staff member may have become more intense either as part of the intensification of treatment, or the increased emphasis on the psychological needs of the patient, or other factors. Having stated the argument we have to say at once that we do not know how important these factors are in the intensification of work load. Dependency studies which are seen as a hopeful development to measure the work load of nurses cannot really take into account the emotional demands on them: their reliability in a comparative study of whether work loads have intensified would be suspect; and even in their obvious use – comparison and measurement of existing work loads – there is a long way to go. 'Ideally there should be a nursing norm – that is, an authoritative set of formulae which, when applied, would indicate the numbers and grades of staff required to provide an agreed standard of nursing care to patients . . . This remains the ultimate objective but the problems which need to be solved before it can be achieved are great.'[14]

In total it is impossible to quantify the impact of these three trends, though they may serve to warn against undue scepticism when faced with complaints about shortages of staff.

On the other side of the coin there have been factors – again unquantifiable – which may have served to reduce pressure on staff. For example, mass production techniques have helped in the provision of disposable instruments and central sterile supplies which have rendered unnecessary some of the jobs of front-line staff. These particular advances must represent considerable gains in available time, especially for nurses. Again, other changes in organisation such as the plating of meals by kitchen staff, addressograph systems and 'topping up' of stores have left front-line staffs more time for their professional duties by reducing the amount of laborious clerical work previously expected of them. And these in turn have been supplemented by improved methods suggested by work study. Although it is impossible to quantify the effect of these improvements, clearly they give the opportunity to increase productivity of front-line personnel. An alternative policy (if it had been feasible) of providing many more personnel may have reduced the effort to find ways to improve productivity.

Another way in which the whole service has been particularly favoured is the probable recruitment of an increasing share of the working population who have received higher education. Mr Bonham Carter, speaking at the 20th Anniversary Conference of the National Health Service pointed out that the public sector in 1964 employed 25 per cent of the labour force and this included

60 per cent of those who had received higher education.[15] No doubt the health services have benefited from this trend, although the standards of performance in the State registration examinations for nursing showed some signs of faltering towards the end of the 1960s.[16] So the health service has not only absorbed an increasing percentage of the labour force but has probably taken a disproportionate share of those of a higher academic calibre.

IV HAVE SHORTAGES OF STAFF BEEN SO ACUTE?

Overall, the health service could hardly be expected to have done better than it has in recruiting more staff. The only valid criticism – and therefore legitimate alibi so to speak – is the mal-distribution of staff geographically, and between the glamorous and non-glamorous areas of practice. If this is accepted, the solution is not merely more staff but may lie in firmer central control over individual preferences of choice of area in which to seek employment. On the question of recruitment, for example, there may be other public services which have stronger claims on available trained manpower than does the health service. It is not obvious how the health service could mount a claim for special preference.

It is hard to mount a substantive case that staff shortages have been the obstacle to improvement some would have us believe. The complaints about shortages either of cash or staff or both only serve to divert attention from the most productive way of improving the service – better management.

5

What is an Adequate Service?

I ASSUMPTIONS

The complaints about shortages have a common starting point.
They assume all those who are sick and need medical treatment
should receive it. This assumption owes much to the debate which
led to the introduction of the National Health Service in 1948.
The nationalisation of the hospital services was seen as the only
way to remedy the deficiencies demonstrated by the preparations
for war. For example, in the case of nursing the only question
seemed to be whether 22,000 or 48,000 *more* nurses were required.[1] There is another associated assumption. This is that additional resources could be produced to meet this unmet demand.

Neither of these two assumptions are tenable. We put forward
an alternative perspective on what constitutes an 'adequate
service by first demonstrating the unhelpfulness of these two
assumptions.

II THE BOTTOMLESS PIT OF HEALTH NEED

For practical purposes the potential demand for health care is
infinite. This has been well illustrated by the concept of the clinical
iceberg. The ill-health known and being treated at any one time by
the health service is only a proportion of morbidity in the community. The volume of potential demand is probably very large.
Table 7 illustrates the size of unmet 'need' in a typical general
practice. It explains the reluctance of some general practitioners
to unleash an avalanche of additional demands on their services
which would follow mass screening programmes. These would
also result in additional demands on other community and
hospital services. And this would be on top of the latter's waiting
lists for admission.

Nor would more preventative services help in the long run.
Patients will live longer, and there will be a greater number of
chronically sick and geriatric patients.

Table 7   *The 'clinical iceberg': estimates of unrecognised disease in an average general practice of 2,250 patients*

	Known	Unknown
Hypertension: males aged 45 +	8	22 Casual diastolic
females aged 45 +	24	107 B.P. 100 mm. Hg. plus
Urinary infection: females 15 +	25	115 Significant bacteriuria
Glaucoma	3	24 Early chronic
Epilepsy	8	6
Diabetes	8	8
Bronchitis: males 45–64	24	24
Rheumatoid arthritis: 15 +	11	14
Psychiatric disorders: males	32	29
females	72	72

Source: Dr J. M. Last (1963), *Lancet*, ii. 28. Quoted in Forsyth, *Doctors and State Medicine: A study of the British Health Service* (Pitman Medical, London 1966), p. 64.

There is another type of unmet demand on particular sectors of the service. There are people who, on medical criteria, require admission to hospital now but whose names are not put on the waiting list for admission. This was forcibly brought home to the author when he was administratively responsible for a group waiting list for admission into chronic sick and geriatric hospitals. The waiting list persisted at about the fifty mark. A new unit for the chronic sick and geriatrics, originally intended to replace existing ex-poor law accommodation, gave the group the opportunity to increase the number of available beds. Some of the poor law beds which were originally intended to be closed were retained. The group waiting list virtually disappeared for three months or so. At the end of that time it began to creep up again. Soon it again hovered about the fifty mark. As one general practitioner cheerfully remarked: 'Before there were patients we didn't bother to put on the waiting list because their priority would be too low. Now we can put them on the waiting list with a reasonable expectation of them being admitted.'

There is another side to this argument. Many would point to the in-patients who do not need the complex and expensive services of a modern hospital, and this is true of a surprisingly high proportion of cases. In one study it was estimated, for example, that 25 per cent of the patients in male medical wards need not have been admitted, if only clinical criteria had been applied; the corresponding figure for females was even higher at 42 per cent.[3] In an ideal world where this was not so, however, these patients would be making some demands on community services. What would be achieved would thus be a redistribution, not a diminution, of workloads. It would add up, too, to an exponential increase in demand for community services. And one could be forgiven for scepticism about the willingness of the hospital services to divert funds to compensate!

The insatiable nature of the health services is dramatically illustrated by an example drawn from the United States. In 1967 a report on manpower resources in the previous year for the American Hospitals Association indicated a total employment of 1,332,000 professional and technical employees. It concluded that 'an increase of 19·3 per cent in the number was necessary to provide optimum patient care . . .'. By 1969 a number of state-wide manpower surveys conducted by state hospital associations and state departments of health reported that 'the staffing levels for most occupational categories had surpassed the level reported to be necessary in 1966 for the delivery of optimal patient care'. Not surprisingly 'by 1969 the manpower requirements for the provision of optimal patient care had increased'.[4] There was still a shortage of staff to meet 'need'.

Concealed morbidity: secondary prevention and survival for further illnesses; unmet need as revealed by waiting lists; and people who are known to general practitioners to be in need but are unable to obtain the right (and often more expensive) treatment together add up to an enormous pool of unmet need. It is so large that its satisfaction is beyond the realm of practical politics. Any conceivable increase in resources will not provide an adequate service. It will merely move the water line a little further down the iceberg.

III   THE UNAVAILABILITY OF ADDITIONAL RESOURCES

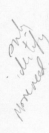

Any concept of adequacy (even in modified form), which would satisfy those running the services would clearly require a large increase in resources. These are unlikely to be forthcoming. This is not merely due to a dislike of higher taxation. Sir Bruce Fraser has pointed out that on occasions in the past the budget surplus has been roughly equal to what we spent on the health service.[5] There are constraints on the amount of money which can be allocated to the National Health Service over and above the willingness and the ability of the taxpayer to pay. Questions of economic management, the claims of other public services, and logistic problems (e.g. are people available to be recruited?) play their part.

Sir Stephen Lycett Green, chairman of the East Anglian Regional Hospital Board, seemed to be facing up to this latter problem towards the end of the last decade. 'The Board hoped to complete three new district hospitals by the end of the 1970s. Estimates prepared in 1965 have shown that these hospitals would require increases of staff of 40 per cent for nursing, 37 per cent for technical staff, 40 per cent for junior medical and 17 per cent over those already in post.'

He felt it was 'unrealistic' to expect them to be recruited from East Anglia.[6] One might be forgiven for thinking he could hardly expect to recruit them elsewhere either; or if he succeeded, whether those in the service would regard it as adequate for long.

If the 'bodies' were available there would be no overwhelming case for them to be diverted to the health services. As far as medical manpower is concerned, one commentator has felt it necessary to point out that 'often social institutions besides medicine have a claim on the available pool of talent from which doctors are recruited. It is possible that medicine already receives its fair share.'[7] And within the health service perhaps the acute hospitals in particular have already been given more than their fair share. If there was a sudden windfall of resources there would be no overwhelming reason why the health services should claim particular priority, or an obvious case for the acute hospitals from which many of the complaints stem, to have priority over other parts of the service.

IV AN ALTERNATIVE PERSPECTIVE ON ADEQUACY

What then is left of the concept of an adequate service? It may be asked, if there are no absolute standards for practical purposes, why then are there so many complaints from those in the service about resources?

Clearly there is a gap between the expectations of those who provide the service and the standard of provision. The problem lies in the staff's belief that their concept of what constitutes an adequate service is a more legitimate one than that held by those who control the resources. No doubt they feel their judgement is sounder because they are so much more aware of the service which the patient actually receives. In fact it is as appropriate for the ultimate controllers of resources, in this case the government, to seek legitimacy for their decision elsewhere – from the taxpayers. And they seem satisfied.[8] Since there is no other obvious way to assess what is adequate, the standard of service for which the consumer is willing to pay and a judgement by the government of its relative importance compared with many other demands on resources must be a prime determinant of what priority should be given to the health service. If this is accepted it is hard to see the intellectual grounds for complaint about shortages, either in 1948 or since.

This is not to say the staff's concept of what constitutes an adequate service is irrelevant. The resources made available must satisfy three groups. First, the consumers; second, the personnel in the service, otherwise their discontent would seriously disrupt it; and third, the government who have to balance the interests of consumers and staff. Indeed, one senior member of the hospital service in the United States has argued the recognition of this potential conflict is in the best interests of the patient. 'Our chief of medicine contends, and I agree with him, that if the doctor tries to economise in the care of patients, he's going to be in real trouble . . . I think you've got to have conflict . . . between the two, of the doctor struggling for the very best for his patient and the people in the hospital struggling for what is possible.'[9]

The desire to improve service is obviously an important feature of professionalism and must be encouraged. The debate, however, will be a fruitful one if those in the service accept

(1) that their expectations will always be higher than the prevailing standards, and thus constitute a claim on future resources rather than what is proper now;
(2) that the absence of resources to meet these higher expectations is 'normal' and does not constitute substantive evidence for charges of unfairness, shortages, etc.;
(3) that the objective of improved services within existing budgets will not be realised until managers accept the *legitimacy* of meeting these aspirations from more efficient use of *present* resources.

This view of the disputes about resources is more constructive than the one which continually emphasises the turpitude, or ignorance, or plain neglect of all governments of the health services. Its acceptance is crucial to any scheme to improve managerial performance.

6

Adequacy and the Responsibility of Health Service Managers

Criticisms of unfair treatment of the health services take up valuable time and energy of people who ought to be doing something more productive. It is not only time and energy: the feeling of unjustness, coupled with the notion of improvements primarily financed by the increment is too ready an excuse for inactivity.

The obvious implication is that the manager must accept that he must first look for other ways of improving the service. There is no doubt in the opinion of at least one ex-minister that the emphasis on shortage is a block to increased efficiency.

A corollary and concomitant of the assumption in an Exchequer-financed service that improvement and progress depend on the Exchequer providing more money is the tendency to neglect and depreciate other sources of betterment. In fact, the diversion of proportionately more effort and resources to an activity is rarely observed to have been a cause of improvement in standards or efficiency, though it has not infrequently been a result . . .[1]

An appreciation of the financial background is an essential prerequisite for the manager at all levels. Blaming superiors for shortage because they have not allocated funds may be a convenient way of releasing one's aggressive feelings; it must not, however, be an automatic excuse for non-improvement of service or passing the buck. Supervisors must not readily accept such explanations as a good reason for being unable to introduce an improvement. And this applies to all who control resources from ward, departmental or district level to the consultant or top administrators. An understanding of the nature of financial constraints hopefully opens the gateway to a greater concentration on the effective use of existing resources. A good manager understands and helps his subordinates to understand.

What can be done to eliminate this defence mechanism? It must

43

somehow be made clear to those in the service that too great an identification with the goal of adequacy is a bar to improvement.

The accomplishment by an administrative programme of its organisational goals can be measured in terms of *adequacy* (the degree to which goals have been reached) or of *efficiency* (the degree to which the goals have been reached relative to the available resources) ... From these two facts (human wants insatiable/no one concept of adequacy) we may conclude that the fundamental criteria of administrative decision must be a criterion of *efficiency* rather than the criterion of *adequacy*. The task of the administrator is to maximise social values *relative* to limited resources.[2] (*My emphasis.*)

Powell seemed to think such a change of emphasis was unlikely in the hospital service because of the system of central financing. This made it 'a positive ethical duty to besiege and bombard the government and force or shame them into providing more money, and then more again ... In these circumstances it is not mendicancy but contentment that would be a crime.'[3]

Where there is a more direct link between those who provide the service and the taxpayers, for example, in local authorities a different atmosphere prevailed. 'They do not run their services down: they praise them and though they recognise deficiencies and objectives still far from being attained, they recognise them as stimuli and incentives, not as material for moaning.'[4]

The new N.H.S. will follow more closely the model of the pre-reform hospital service. The change of emphasis from adequacy to efficiency has to be effected with the system which Powell regarded as an insuperable obstacle to that change firmly *in situ*.

Opportunities to obtain additional resources for development from the existing allocations still exist. For example, Butterworth has reported a study in two large hospitals which suggested that output could be (and was) increased by 20 to 30 per cent by reorganisation of methods. Another illustration was a hospital where six out of thirteen vehicles in the transport fleet were sold or not replaced.[5] Even in the difficult area of junior medical staff's working hours, improvements can be made without necessarily requiring additional expenditure. A study at Victoria Hospital, Kirkcaldy, of the work undertaken by registrars, senior house officers and house officers at night and at weekends indicated that sufficient cover could be provided by keeping four house officers on duty rather than the six or seven who had been previously required. Admittedly the change produced a heavier workload for those on duty and the additional problem of more cross coverage between specialties. But in return it was possible to arrange a substantial increase in off-duty time.[6] These are but a few examples of how additional resources for improvements can be made available without waiting for additional resources. We give more examples later.

On a much broader front Feldstein's study of 177 acute non-teaching hospitals gives us some idea of the room for improvement. He found that about one-third of inter-hospital variations in cost per case could be explained by case mix differences.[7] No doubt there are factors other than efficiency which explain some of the remaining variations. But there is little doubt that different levels of efficiency within the hospital sector accounted for a substantial amount of the discrepancy. This gives some idea of the substantial scope for improvement in some of the weaker hospitals. Clearly, the resources which could be made available for improvement by more efficiency are greater than any reasonable expectation of what the increment might provide. The management problem, then, is to increase efforts to find these additional resources and to make them the *legitimate* way to finance improvements.

We discuss efficient management and its implications in Chapters 12 to 19. However, three general points merit a mention at this stage. First, shortages of staff are often measured by the number of unfilled vacancies within the approved establishment. If there is no sure way of saying what is an adequate number of staff, what, one might ask, are the value of establishment figures? Is the work which has been done, for example, on formulae to calculate the required number of nurses pointless? They are not pointless if regarded, for example, as *claims* on future resources or a means of setting priorities for development. As management tools establishments are invaluable: it is when the establishment figures are regarded as inalienable rights they are a source of inefficiency.

Second, there is the question of control of expenditure. At the respiratory unit at St Thomas's there would have been considerable difficulties if the additional demand was not met; similarly with the prescriptions for L. Dopa. Yet clearly not all additional demand can be met. No ward unit, district or hospital is an island. One ward's overspending can be another department's planned improvement. Expenditure can be increased almost imperceptibly. Where this happens, conscious decisions on priorities can be overturned. It is an implication of this argument that in a system which gives greater emphasis to efficiency there must be more open acknowledgment of the fact of rationing: all demand is not and cannot be met.

It follows that the claims of a new 'demand' on resources must first be measured against other priorities: it must not automatically pre-empt funds allocated for planned improvements. Such decisions cannot be left to individual units or clinicians: one man's overspending is another's improvement. Such an approach requires conscious decisions on priorities by teams of officers.

Third, there is the question of impact on the morale of personnel in the service. Some have attributed low morale among at least hospital staff partly to the belief that the service has been inadequately financed.[8] Given that resources will always be less than people in the service feel to be adequate, what can managers do about these feelings of unfairness which might in turn have an adverse impact on morale? They must maintain morale by accepting and explaining the economic facts of life. Acquiescence or agreements with complaints about shortage will not produce more resources or improve the service. It follows that if morale plummets among staff because of beliefs about shortages, at least in the more favoured sectors of the service, then the responsibility is mainly that of the local managers. They must seek to scale down unrealistic expectations of providers by education. It is a sign of an inefficient manager if he encourages them.

The general implications for managers in the health service are clear. They must make better use of existing resources to obtain the margin for improvement. It is inefficient to wait for the increment before introducing change without first examining existing commitments and levels of efficiency. It is inefficient to allow expectations to leap ahead of likely provision. It is inefficient not to acknowledge that other sectors of public expenditure, or of the health service may not have a greater priority. It is inefficient to find refuge from challenging decisions in complaints about inadequacy.

Such an argument may sound idealistic. Certainly the years of preaching by ministers and civil servants seem not to have produced a change in attitude towards resources among some key personnel. Does the commitment to the best regardless of cost and the effect of dependence on central finance produce so formidable a barrier that such a change in approach is impossible? Only time will tell whether the intensive courses in management training are sufficient to offset them, and produce a greater emphasis on efficiency.

7
Organisation and the Manager

I THE DISADVANTAGES OF THE OLD STRUCTURE

Shortages were one alibi for the manager who wished to divert attention from his own responsibilities for slow or non-development of services. Another was the form of organisation chosen for the health service in 1948. The structure was believed to have imposed three very serious constraints on the manager.

Firstly, the division of responsibilities between the executive councils, local health authorities and the hospital service made effective co-ordination between them difficult. Secondly, the absence of a 'scientific' management structure in the hospital service produced a lack of direction, uncertainties about responsibilities and consequently a less than optimum use of resources. And thirdly, the requirements of public finance and the consequent emphasis on propriety of expenditure made for difficulties in the flexible and more effective use of funds.

These criticisms were widely accepted and indeed largely explain the 1974 reform. They have to be seen, however, against a background of widespread dissatisfaction with the way our public services are organised. Very few parts of the public sector have been spared the trauma of reorganisation in the last decade or so. It is now the turn of the health service.

It is not part of our brief to discuss the case for the reform of the service. Our interest is much more specific. We are concerned with the relationship between the formal structure of the service and the everyday management problems of those who run it. We are concerned to identify those features of organisation which are a hindrance to the manager and those which facilitate his attempts to improve the service. We shall also try to identify those factors which precipitate breakdowns and will thus remain problem areas for the manager.

The three criticisms of the old structure provide the context for this exploration. In this chapter we discuss the contribution of the division of responsibilities between different authorities to the

47

breakdowns in co-ordination at grass roots level. The second and third criticisms are discussed in the subsequent two chapters.

II   THE TRIPARTITE STRUCTURE OF THE HEALTH SERVICES: THE ESSENTIALS OF GOOD CO-ORDINATION

We begin by first establishing what we mean by optimal co-ordination. This is best done by way of example. We have chosen the discharge from hospital of an elderly patient who requires an ambulance. We pick up the story after the patient's suitability for discharge has already been settled. This process of course will already have included assessment of home conditions preferably by a medical social worker. The point of the exercise is to ensure the delivery of the right service in the right sequence at the right time.

A well co-ordinated service will ensure that:

(1) Maximum notice of the date of discharge is given to the patient.
(2) Information on the discharge is given to relatives.
(3) Necessary community services have been

   (a) arranged (not merely informed);
   (b) been given sufficient medical and social information to perform their functions efficiently,
   (c) told the date and time of discharge.

(4) The ambulance department have been requested to provide transport in good time and they have been informed of the time and place from which the patient is to be discharged; the kind of vehicle which would be most suitable and the address to which the patient is to be taken.

   It might also be necessary to confirm that suitable arrangements have been made.

(5) The patient and/or his relatives are told of all these arrangements. This is particularly important if the relatives are going to be closely involved in arrangements for the reception and care of the patient on discharge.
(6) The patient is told clearly with supplementation in written form what the next steps in the treatment process will be.

No doubt readers can think of other important steps which should be taken but this broad outline is sufficient for our purposes.

There are two elements which ensure the success of an operation of this type. First, strict adherence to procedures where these exist. Routine procedures are appropriate where the activity involved is a frequent one. They ensure consistency in the way arrangements are made. The behaviour of fellow workers is predictable. Since the procedures are frequently used they are easily remembered and initiated with little effort.

Where patients are involved there are many occasions where established routines are not wholly appropriate. Some unusual factor will arise and arrangements made accordingly. These necessitate *ad hoc* decisions which in turn require an accurate assessment of the availability of other services and their likely response to the request for assistance.

An illustration perhaps helps to make the distinction clearer. It is in fact a slightly modified account of an actual case. A nurse had broken her ankle and had been X-rayed at a general practitioner hospital some fifteen miles from her home. It was agreed that she could return home but she would need to see the consultant orthopod at the district general hospital in a third town. The district general hospital was approximately equidistant from the nurse's home town and the general practitioner unit. The general practitioner had suggested that the ambulance service be asked to make a detour of some ten to twelve miles between the nurse's home and the district general hospital to collect the X-rays for the consultant. On this basis the out-patient appointment was made.

In this case routine procedures for fixing transport and the out-patient appointment were insufficient to ensure the whole operation ran smoothly. They had to be supplemented by special, *ad hoc* arrangements to ensure the X-rays were collected and delivered to the consultant orthopod. The arrangements which were made assumed a particular response from the ambulance service. This is the element of judgement about the likely response of fellow workers which characterises the second important element in good co-ordination. In this particular case the judgement was wrong. The ambulance service refused to do the detour.

Most of the arrangements made for the discharge of our elderly patient would fall within the category of routine procedures. For example, it would be specified (in an ideal situation) who decided the necessity for community services and which particular ones were required; the method of informing these services and the type and content of the communication; the means of ordering an ambulance; and when and by whom the patient and relatives should be told what has been arranged and what happens next. *Ad hoc* arrangements clearly may be required to supplement these procedures thus requiring judgement of the response of other services. Problems of co-ordination arise from failure to follow procedures and from faulty judgement of the needs and responses of fellow employees.

In what ways did the division of responsibilities between the three arms of the service cause or contribute to these failings? There is little doubt that there were frequent breakdowns. Examples were legion. The most popular ones were those involving hospitals discharging non-ambulant patients to an empty house with little or no notice to community services; hospitals being asked to do jobs which were properly the job of the general practitioner or community services; the general practitioner ordering home helps who did not arrive: the seeming impossibility of co-ordinating ambulance journeys to get patients to out-patient departments or day centres at the specified times. Or the slowness of the laboratory or the X-ray department in responding to urgent requests for investigation and report. In one study of the experience of patients discharged from hospital it was found that within a period of two weeks 'the number of community workers called upon to help was double those arranged by hospital staff'.[1]

It is not always clear from the literature and the reports which of the two factors were responsible for these 'horror' stories. No doubt on occasions it was because routine procedures had not been established or, if they had been established, not adhered to. The failure of hospital medical staff to write to general practitioners until a considerable time after the patient's discharge would be an example of this. No doubt on other occasions it was because the needs and responses of other services had been incorrectly appraised and the anticipated response had not been forthcoming.

An assumption that these failures and the division of responsibilities are related does not tell us much about the specific factors which caused the trouble. We need now to look at a specific case to help us identify some of them.

III   THE CASE OF THE RELUCTANT AMBULANCE SERVICE

The case concerned a cantankerous man in his late sixties. He lived in lodgings, and had no relatives in the area. The general practitioner felt that his patient should be admitted to a geriatric hospital for the care which he was unlikely to get in the rather unsatisfactory conditions in which he lived. When the man indicated that he would not agree to go into hospital the medical officer of health and a county welfare officer agreed that he should be compulsorily admitted.

The hospital management committee kept a group waiting list for admission to its three geriatric hospitals, all of which were in different towns. The hospital in the town in which the man lived had only two male beds. The county welfare officer, as was usual, contacted the group officer responsible for the waiting list. There was a good working relationship at this level. The welfare officers readily understood if they were told a case of this type was not as urgent as others on the list and delayed the application for the order. If the welfare officers, who did some domiciliary visiting and fact-finding at the request of the group officer, said a case was very urgent this judgement was accepted equally readily.

The patient was duly admitted by a hospital 17 miles from the town in which he lived, and in which the magistrate's court was located. As the expiry date of the order drew near he was visited by the medical officer of health and county welfare officer. After consultations with the hospital medical officer, it was agreed that the patient was not yet fit enough for discharge or transfer to local authority welfare accommodation. On being so informed the patient again indicated he would not stay voluntarily. He was not surprisingly told an application would therefore be made for a new court order. This time, however, the patient said he wanted to be present at the hearing to contest it. The medical officer of health undertook to arrange the transport to meet the patient's wishes. On returning to his office, the medical officer informed the ambulance service of the transport required.

The first sign of a problem came when the ambulance department asked the hospital secretary whether the management committee would pay for the cost of transporting the man to and from the hospital for the hearing. Since the ambulance was based in the town where the magistrate's court was held, this would involve four journeys, totalling at least sixty-eight miles. There was also the problem of waiting time at the court. While the debate between the hospital staff and the hospital management committee went on as to whether the hospital service could or should take on this responsibility, fresh attempts were made by the welfare officer and the medical officer of health to persuade the ambulance department to provide the transport at no cost. It should be added that the ambulance department was very helpful about transferring patients between hospitals when asked to do so by the group administrator in charge of the geriatric waiting lists. Clearly some of these journeys did *not* come within the scope of the National Health Service Act but no account was raised by the ambulance department. Provided such requests were made with discretion there was no question of payment. Yet a request (admittedly out of the ordinary) from the colleagues of the ambulance officer led to a refusal.

In the event, the treasurer of the hospital management committee ruled that such charges could not be met out of the exchequer funds; requests to samaritan funds, and voluntary organisations attached to the hospital produced no substantive response. The magistrate's clerk felt they had no funds to meet such a case; likewise the National Assistance Board. The ambulance officer of the County Council asked the treasurer for a ruling as to whether he should provide the service. To nobody's surprise this answer too was in the negative. The man had insufficient funds to finance the journeys himself.

In this case the primary breakdown was within the *same* authority. The medical officer accepted responsibility and ordered the ambulance; it was the ambulance service who voiced the objections. The medical officer of health who had committed himself to the provision of ambulance transport for the man was clearly embarrassed.

The relationships between the management committee and the ambulance officer in contrast seemed much more relaxed. There was a mutual confidence across organisational boundaries which permitted limited favours. And this persisted over time in spite of changes of personnel.

IV CO-ORDINATION BETWEEN AUTHORITIES

Where does this very unusual case lead us? Most obviously it suggests that breakdowns are not exclusively caused by a division of responsibility between separate authorities. Co-ordination between the separate authorities was good. Levine and White's analysis of inter-organisational relationships helps us to understand why this might be so.

They have suggested that co-ordination can be understood as a system of exchanges between organisations.[2] Resources (e.g. information, personnel and finance) are exchanged to help both organisations achieve their goals. Three types of inter-organisational relationship have been suggested – independent (not applicable to our analysis but included for completeness), interdependence, and conflict.

In the case study an interdependent relationship existed between the management committee officer on the one hand and with the ambulance department and the county welfare officer on the other.

The relationship with the ambulance service was typified by the care taken to ensure early notifications of requests for transport, thus permitting the ambulance officer to plan ahead, and only asking a minimum of favours. The nature of the cases too allowed considerable notice of the need for transport. The ambulance service was thus left with considerable discretion to plan their work. This in turn made it easier for the ambulance service to meet their objectives of maximising the use of ambulances and give the management committee a reliable, dependable service. The good co-ordination which can flow from interdependence and which in turn helps both parties to meet their objectives was apparent in this particular relationship.

It might be argued that the area health board structure makes this high level of interdependence the norm rather than the exception since both the service seekers and service givers will be in the same integrated authority. If so, presumably many of the problems of co-ordination, for example, between the hospital and ambulance staff will be resolved. This is probably too optimistic a view as another possibility remains – a conflict relationship. The ambulance service will still be under pressure to maximise the use of their fleet of vehicles. But they will now be in direct competition with other health service staff, with whom they will be in a service relationship, for resources, political power and status. In such a situation co-operation may sometimes be less forthcoming than in this case study and co-ordination may become *more* difficult! It might be argued that White and Levine's analysis refers to relationships between organisations, and is therefore inappropriate as a basis for analysing the integrated structure. Yet in a large organisation, as the area health authority will inevitably be, boundary exchanges between departments will clearly retain some of the characteristics of inter-organisational ones.

It follows from this too that an important element in successful co-ordination is the quality of management. Resourceful managers can overcome these obstacles. There were many examples of well-developed integrated services across the tripartite boundaries before 1974. At Doncaster the domiciliary midwives of the County Borough were employed by the hospital management committee and the domiciliary service run from the hospital maternity department. Domiciliary midwives also helped in the wards and delivery rooms.[3]

Another example was a scheme for early discharge and out-patient surgery at the Western General Hospital, Edinburgh, which involved twenty-eight general practitioners and nineteen district nurses. The latter participated in the pre-operative selection and post-operative care. Between 1967 and 1970 this co-operative scheme had seen over 600 patients managed in this way and more than 2,000 bed days saved. Only a low incidence of complications was reported among the first fifty discharges.[4] These are but two of the many examples of excellent inter-organisational co-operation.

Where there is this high degree of co-operation our second requirement for good co-ordination is more easily met. The response and needs of other staff to requests for co-operation will be more accurately anticipated. Even within authorities, as our case study demonstrates, this is not guaranteed!

So far we have warned against unrealistic expectations of the beneficial impact of integration on the everyday problems of the manager and against uncritical acceptance of the notion that the tripartite structure was the major obstacle to co-ordination on the ground. Yet reform clearly will help. It will provide, hopefully, a point to which problems can be referred for adjudication without involving the Department as hitherto. More importantly it might provide more concordance between the objectives of the various parts of the service. And since these objectives will guide the responses of personnel in the service, it should be easier to predict them when *ad hoc* arrangements have to be made to ensure delivery of a co-ordinated service.

8

Co-ordination within Authorities: the Experience of the Hospital Service

I THE OFFICIAL DIAGNOSIS

The factors which were held to be responsible for difficulties in co-ordinating hospital services are clear in the prescriptions for the management structure for the new service. In short, it was the absence of a clear management structure. Sir Keith Joseph, in the foreword to the Consultative Document on Reorganisation emphasised the need for drawing clear lines of responsibility and accountability throughout the levels of authority.[1] And Professor Elliot Jaques, whose ideas were clearly influential in the proposals for the management structure of the new authorities agrees. 'Why all this emphasis on organisation? Because, in my view, unless we can get our organisations clarified, described, formulated, understood, we are not going to be able to make any fundamental progress towards systematic and effective management.'[2]

For many, the criticisms of the management structure, and its responsibility for management difficulties, have a more specific focus. It is the absence of a supreme boss which is seen as the basic cause of breakdowns. These critics would point to the ambulance case study and say the problem would have been solved if there had been one central point where responsibilities could be clarified and a solution imposed. It is often felt that if only there was a supreme being who was invested with the authority to enforce his will, and to whom staff could appeal, all would be well. Obviously some hospital administrators feel this to be so. In *The Shape of Hospital Management in 1980*, for example, there was a recommendation that a district hospital general manager be appointed. S. G. Hill, in his contribution to *Modern Hospital Management* saw the administrator playing this role. He distinguishes between the administrative content of every job and the administration of the entire hospital which is, however, a much bigger and wider thing, which must be the sole responsibility of the administrator'.[3] But what contribution to improved co-ordination would the supreme being make? Even Mr MacIver, to whose ideas we have already referred, would not see the general manager in a sufficiently authoritative position to co-ordinate forcibly. He sees the consultant, for example, as a functional specialist, and it is only when they operate outside their own function 'must they operate through line management'.[4] In such an organisation the problems of getting the medical, engineering, catering, portering, nursing staff, etc. to co-ordinate their services with one's own would remain. The existence of 'functional specialists' makes a strategy of co-ordination by the structural authority of a supreme being neither effective nor likely.

This is so whether the general manager is a doctor or layman. This topic is a well-rehearsed one among those faced with the problems of co-ordinating their services with others. It assumes that the prestige of the doctor, and his identification with what is thought to be the primary goal of the hospital, will be sufficient to ensure co-operation and thus improve co-ordination. A personal experience will perhaps suffice to throw doubts on this view. A group secretary had arranged with the physician superintendent that I, as a management trainee, should spend some time in the operating theatre unit. It was agreed that I should observe operations. I arrived on the appointed day to be informed by the theatre superintendent that the surgeons had decided I should not watch operations. The physician superintendent's writ did not run as far as the surgeons. This is a good example of badly co-ordinated training for a student. Arrangements had been made for the attachment because it was assumed that certain experiences would be available. Only after misunderstandings based on the different expectations of the participants of what was to be provided was the author told of the decision. The physician superintendent had neither the authority to ensure there were no such breakdowns nor to put them right. A member of the medical staff is as unlikely as a general lay administrator – even if he were helped by the formal designation as head of the organisation – to co-ordinate other staff forcibly.

However, the case for clarification of lines of authority, responsibility and accountability is a separate issue. Support for this position does not imply support for a single general manager.

A substantial body of opinion regards a much more 'scientific' management structure as crucial in the integrated service. It is the view, as we have said, of the Secretary of State and the Brunel researchers. It was the view too of the Salmon Committee, the committee which produced the Cogwheel report as well as contributors to the book, *Modern Hospital Management*. There are many others who have voiced the same view. The advantages are not confined to co-ordination, which is the particular aspect of management which we have chosen to discuss. It is also felt to facilitate greater emphasis on accountable management. And Mr MacIver has argued that 'the adoption of Urwick's principle of definition would have prevented misunderstandings, stresses and struggles for position . . .'[5]

In the particular context of co-ordination it is pointed out that if we can decide the two questions: (a) who is responsible for what? and (b) what exactly does this responsibility entail? staff will have clear expectations of their own role and that of others. Provided responsibilities are matched with commensurate authority problems of co-ordination should then be less.

It is easy to overestimate the effect of this kind of reform on the day-to-day problems of co-ordination. In such a system the laboratory technician will be quite clear about the correct response to the junior doctor who has asked for a test requiring the approval of a consultant. He will not do it. Clear definition of one's responsibilities in, for example, a job description, makes it quite clear for what things one is *not* responsible and therefore *not* expected to do. The junior doctor hopefully will in future go through the correct channels and not exceed his authority. He will also correctly anticipate the technician's refusal to do the test.

We must beware of over-optimistic assessments of the impact of organisational change on problems of co-ordination. Breakdowns and difficulties have roots which are not amenable to remedies of this type. There are other reasons why the responses and information needs of others are wrongly assessed. Much will depend on the ability of managers to recognise and understand these other causes of difficulties. Taking the pre-reform hospital service as our setting let us now try and identify some of these other causes of breakdown in co-ordination.

II CO-ORDINATION WITHIN AUTHORITIES. OTHER
    CAUSES OF BREAKDOWN

(a) *The problem of uncertainty*
We said in the previous chapter that routine procedures were a way of ensuring good co-ordination. However, in the health services uncertainty about outcomes precludes many routine procedures for co-ordination. This is also the view of Spencer:

'But in hospitals there are no "long runs"; every patient must be treated as a separate entity to which the care has to be tailored. And because the patient's needs may change unpredictably in the course of his treatment, planning can rarely be far ahead and must always be adaptable. Often no mechanical system or formal procedure is feasible.'[6]   Clearly, successful co-ordination in the health services depends much more on a correct appreciation of the needs and responses of other staff than many other organisations. The very complexity of management relationships in the health service, the scope for the pursuit of departmental and personal goals make such appreciations problematic.

(b) Complexity of relationships

The different types of responsibility (and therefore authority and accountability) which are associated with different posts in hospitals have been well illustrated by Packwood.[7] Taking the hospital secretary as an example he argues he can have four qualitatively different relationships with different staff:

(a) As structural superior, e.g. medical records department.
(b) As joint superior, e.g. with group catering officer for the work of hospital catering staff.
(c) As co-ordinator and monitor, e.g. towards engineering staff.
(d) As service seeker, e.g. towards hospital building staff who are asked to provide a service for his department.

Applying these concepts to the nursing staff, a ward sister would have a similarly wide variety of different relationships:

(a) As superior, e.g. nursing auxiliary.
(b) As joint superior, e.g. of cleaning staff on the ward; this responsibility she shares with the domestic superintendent. Where the ward sister's responsibility is clearly 'sapiental' her relationships with domestic or, say, catering staff may be more properly described in (c). Another example of this type of relationship is with student nurses for whose training she has joint responsibility with the nurse training school.
(c) As co-ordinator and monitor, e.g. of services provided by domestic and catering staff on her ward.
(d) As service seeker, e.g. for para-medical services for the patient.

Obviously clarification of functions and responsibilities coupled with management training will enable staff to understand these relationships intellectually and supplement intuitive appreciation of them. Obviously, too, training and education will help them to see their implications. But, given the subtlety and complexity of these different relationships, not all are amenable to 100 per cent clarification or understanding, or to consistent adherence to different behaviours which are implied in them.

This point is strengthened when we acknowledge that so far we have not described the whole range of different relationships in which the sister, for example, is involved. So far we have only mentioned her relationships with junior staff or peers. There are four other relationships in an 'upward' direction, each of a different texture. First, relationships with the medical staff and in particular the consultant. Jaques has described this relationship as characterised by a 'prescriptive authority'. 'He is not the manager of nurses: he is not accountable for their work: he cannot issue instructions to specific individuals.'[8] This description of consultant/nurse relationships may raise a wry smile among some nurses. In one hospital which the author visited in the course of research some sisters (including the young, progressive ones) differentiated between their responsibilities to consultants on the basis of sectors of work rather than by types of relationship. 'In clinical matters the consultant is my boss: the assistant matron is not technically equipped to help me,' was the type of comment heard. There is also the added dimension of the variations in relationships between and within hospitals.

The second upward relationship is with the administrative nursing staff: the third with the hospital administrator and the fourth with her professional association. Even those who would not agree with the universality of Jaques' description of nurse/consultant relationships will agree that there are subtle differences in the texture of these four relationships.

Together they make sufficient demand on the ward sister's evaluative system, without having to appreciate the different textures of relationships with peers and juniors. Front-line managers can be forgiven, particularly when under pressure from the consultant or general practitioner in the case of community nurses, if they adopt an inappropriate posture for a particular relationship. In so doing they provoke an unhelpful response which makes co-ordination more difficult.

An illustration from the author's own experience may make this last point clearer. A theatre sister (there was no superintendent) was told by the pathologist that there was a source of infection in one of the theatre drains and the chemical solution which was required to combat it. Both the sister and the surgeons were understandably anxious for speedy action and she contacted the pharmacist immediately. Her relationship with the pharmacist was clearly that of a service-seeker. However, she was under pressure to act quickly and had been told what to order from the pharmacy. When she made the request she was surprised to be asked what the nature of the infection was; to be told that it was not her job to prescribe or for her to assume that the pathologist knew the most appropriate agent to counter the infection. She did not get the solution for which she asked but what the pharmacist felt was the most appropriate. No doubt the pharmacist informed the pathologist and obtained his consent. In the event little was lost except the time spent debating and listening to the pharmacist's point of view; the procedure for controlling the source of the infection worked well. But the theatre sister had used the wrong posture in a service-seeking relationship, particularly as the request had not been presented in the routine form for the sake of speed. In a less urgent situation one could see such a wrong approach producing obstruction leading to considerable difficulties in co-ordination. In another context it is not difficult to envisage a departmental head adopting an approach more applicable to a superior/inferior relationship to a cleaner and producing the inevitable 'Who does he think he is . . . just wait and see!'

A major cause of breakdown is clearly the sheer complexity of hospital management. Integration is going to add another dimension to that complexity. Clarification does not reduce this complexity. It rather makes the different relationships more intelligible! The demands on one's appreciative system are still great. And we have identified defective appreciation as a source of the misjudgement of the response of others.

(c) *Personalities*

Not all non-co-operation can be ascribed to a wrong appreciation of a particular formal relationship. One is always aware in large organisations of people who seem to make difficulties when asked to provide a service. Where this happens it is often ascribed to personality. 'He's a difficult chap' or 'You know her, she thinks she's Florence.' The formal management structure minimises this problem insofar as it insists on procedures and adherence to them. However, its contribution is minimal where formal procedures are inappropriate.

However, before taking this explanation (or alibi) for poor co-ordination at face value, it is worth reflecting on the frequency with which certain departments have staff who in the view of those seeking a service, are often difficult and unco-operative. Two hospital departments which figure prominently in comments of practitioners to the author are those of the engineer and the pharmacist. Problems of intra-organisational co-ordination often seem to be greater if one of these departments is involved. Repairs considered urgent by ward and department staff do not seem to be given the same priority by maintenance staff. Or requisitions to the pharmacy seem to be frequently queried (Are you eating it?) or sometimes changed. From the viewpoint of these two departments, things naturally seem somewhat different. 'Always waving the shroud' is one response. I well remember pharmacists' tales of what they had found in their inspections of ward drug cupboards – tales told with a mixture of horror, incredulity and relish.

On many management training courses I have offered descriptions of an engineer or pharmacist (and other grades of staff) which students have acknowledged to be a fair description of their own. Yet members came from different hospitals and the descriptions were an amalgam of the various engineers and pharmacists I had met in other parts of the country. Does this not suggest that the explanations for any lack of co-operation cannot entirely be particular personalities? And there are reasons why these and other heads of department respond as they do?

One reason could be an organisational factor. The maintenance engineer has his own priorities – and they may be different from those who seek his service. His major preoccupation is naturally to prevent the breakdown of major plant. Again workmen naturally want to plan their work and are understandably reluctant to do small additional jobs if the time they take to do an assignment is checked or if there is an incentive bonus scheme. Unless, say, the sister who is most concerned about a window in the sluice room which won't quite close understands the pressure on the maintenance department, she will wrongly assess his likely response ('Why doesn't she do it herself? She can wait.'). His different set of priorities can be a mystery to her.

We must see the organisation through the eyes of the other participants. 'Action derives from the meanings that men attach to their own and each other's acts.'[9] We should look more at the reasons for their behaviour, the constraints under which people operate and the ends that individuals pursue in organisations. Only by so doing will staff correctly anticipate the response of a fellow decision-maker to a request and thus maximise the probability of co-operation. An assumption that staff are similarly motivated is dangerous. But what are these ends which might motivate them?

(d) Personal and departmental goals

Burns and Stalker suggest that the behaviour of managers and professionals might be better understood if we acknowledge that not only is a member of staff an employee but 'a member of a group with sectional interest in conflict with other groups' and 'one individual among many to whom the rank they occupy and the prestige attaching to them are matters of deep concern'. Burns and Stalker call the first the 'political' and the second the 'status' system of the concern.[10] Some are prepared to acknowledge this fact of organisational life[11] although one senior member of the hospital service did tell me angrily that 'considerations of status do not arise in hospitals. We only consider the good of the patients.' No doubt she had other explanations for the different sizes of offices, carpets, availability of telephones, etc.

Let us now try to develop and apply these ideas to the engineer and pharmacist. We have said priorities differ and a lack of appreciation of this fact can obviously lead to misunderstandings. But has the engineers' department sectional interests which conflict with those of other groups? What objectives could conflict with those of other departments? The essential problem of the engineers' department is to ration demand on their time and keep the essential services running. One way to cope with the pressures from other staff is to be elusive. And one of the characteristics of the engineer to which many of my students have assented and within my experience is his elusiveness. Even the 'bleep' somehow doesn't produce him. In this way the engineer can more easily pursue the things which he perceives as important. In this way, too, he avoids the necessity of saying 'no' so often to requests from departments. It increases his power over his own workload and over the staff who require his service.

And what of the pharmacist? Motivated by status? What can be more irritating for a university-trained man employed in a pharmaceutical role considered inferior by his peers,[12] to be told by some student nurse that a junior doctor wants X when he knows that there is probably a more effective alternative or a cheaper substitute. Even if this is not so, the minimum requirement for co-operation is to demonstrate the respect due to the pharmacist – 'ask humbly and you will receive; tell him what you want and there will be trouble'.

One strategy to enhance political power and status is to preserve and enlarge areas of discretion. Silverman argues this limits their 'dependence on others' by making future behaviour 'more unpredictable'.[13] This strategy could explain the elusiveness of the engineer. Its everyday use is illustrated by an example from the author's own experience. The hospital secretary had been asked by the group secretary to counter-sign the pharmacist's orders for supplies. This procedure had .been instituted because the pharmacist had once used his purchasing powers to buy some supplies for matron which had been refused by the secretary. This was a matter of indignity for the pharmacist. 'I'm the responsible person – he doesn't know what he's signing for.' His method of underlining this was late delivery of orders to the secretary's office for urgent despatch that night. Either the hospital secretary refused to sign them that night and held up important orders or signed them without scrutiny. Usually he did the latter. Although honour was not quite satisfied the pharmacist had made the point that *he* was responsible and the secretary had no effective jurisdiction over his ordering. Who signs what is an important decision in the perception of the participants, determining or reflecting power and status in an organisation. The pharmacist's response to this procedure *de facto* maintained his area of discretion, and demonstrated his independence, power and status in the organisation.

There are perhaps other personal goals which, if unrecognised by colleagues, will lead to an incorrect prediction of likely response. One such goal which deserves mention is that of personal satisfaction. A children's nurse, for example, may have chosen that role because she liked children to be dependent on her. This might have been truer in the past when there were more unmarried women who did not have the opportunity to have their own children. For a nurse who was so motivated the increased pressure to permit and encourage the mother to visit frequently and in certain circumstances stay overnight in hospital may not have been altogether welcome. It would be difficult to put forward the personal needs of nurses (if they were recognised) as a counter-argument. The arguments about infection and the genuine intellectual doubts about the actual effect of separation were important strands in the resistance of nursing staff to this development. But this desire to have children dependent on her ('they don't bring them up properly anyway') may also have been important.

In what ways could we say this, if it be true, produced breakdowns in co-ordination? It could explain, for example, why management instructions were so often not carried out in the spirit they were intended. In one children's hospital in which the author was involved in a research capacity the leaflet to parents stated quite clearly that parents could visit any time, although the hours between which it would be more convenient to come were also given. The management committee and the regional hospital board were assured by the senior officers that 'free' visiting was allowed. After all, they had asked that it be so. In fact, in one of the wards parents who came to visit before the 'convenient' time were kept behind a gate on the stairs. The gate was unlocked during those hours between which the management committee had said it was most convenient to visit. Parents were told one thing, but the sister did not behave in a way consistent with this information. The management committee wrongly estimated the response of the sister on this particular ward. We do not know what motivated the sister to do this. What we do know is that she interpreted a particular policy so that it was more consistent with what she wanted. A possible motive was the personal need to which we referred. The net result was inconvenience and confusion for parents.

These objectives (personal satisfaction, political status) contribute to bad co-ordination if fellow decision-makers assume others are not motivated by them, or wrongly assess their commitment to them. Some feel that these personal objectives exist but are less important in services like the health service. 'What does follow from the nature of the hospitals work and the emotional involvement of its staff is that the goals of the individual members and the objectives of the organisations are much more likely to coincide than they do in other organisations.'[14] Perhaps, but the scandals in our long-stay hospitals in the last five or six years should warn us against too optimistic a view.

The position is further complicated by the different objectives of the service. The emphasis given to a particular objective (cure, care, staff satisfaction, training) differs between staff. It is not always obvious what the 'normal' response to a request is going to be in an untypical situation. It may be that since objectives are unclear 'personal' motives play a bigger part in decisions in the health service than we would like to admit.

We may have given the impression that the pursuit of such objectives is a personal affair. If so, we have to emphasise these types of goals are often shared by members of a department or a professional group. Identification with interests of a subgroup, department or particular hospital is a well-established phenomena. Responses to requests for service are partly conditioned by a desire to protect and further the group's interests. It is via the group that the individual can further his own objectives. Striving for professional status as well as the protection of the interests of other members of the occupational group falls into this typology. As with personal goals the political and status objectives of a department will be couched in acceptable terms. 'It will be in the interests of the patient if such and such a function is transferred to my department,' etc.

It goes without saying that such objectives are rarely articulated. Political, status, personal interests stated as baldly as this are hardly acceptable currency in any welfare institution. They have to be pursued in more oblique ways. 'It would be in the interests of efficiency to have an engineer directly responsible to the Board.' A place at the top table is a phrase which has gained currency in another context. In the hospital context, claims by treasurers, engineers, matrons, pharmacists, etc. to have a place at the top table are often examples of what we have labelled 'personal goals' at work. These factors, as Spencer suggests, may be less important in the health services than in non-welfare organisations.[15] On the other hand they may be enhanced by the lack of specific organisational objectives by which one can judge the correctness of one's decision and by the proportion of decisions that cannot be reduced to a routine procedure to ensure automatic co-ordination.

It is the lack of awareness of these factors in one's own behaviour ('I think only of the patient') and that of others that leads to a wrong assessment of the needs and likely responses of fellow decision-makers.

The absence of a sound management structure in a hospital service may have made a difficult situation more difficult. Without clear objectives with which to identify and which can be assumed to determine the response of others there will be misunderstandings. These will not be eliminated by organisational reform. The quality of management is at least, if not more, important.

III AN APPROACH TO MANAGEMENT IN THE NEW SERVICE

An obvious implication of our argument so far is a cautious approach to changes in formal arrangements as a means of solving management problems. There are other reasons to take this standpoint.

One of the most important is the rapid changes in demand and technology. Changes in demand coupled with the introduction of new treatments and new equipment combine to make routines outmoded, and raise new problems for which no established procedures are particularly appropriate.

In a study of the electronics industry, Burns and Stalker found there were similar difficulties in predicting the volume and the nature of future work load.[16] In these circumstances what they called a 'mechanistic' system of management, which sought to regulate interaction by clearly defined procedures was unhelpful. 'In mechanistic systems of management the problems and tasks facing the concern as a whole are broken down into specialisms. Each individual pursues his task . . . as if it were the subject of a sub-contract . . . The technical methods, duties and powers attached to each functional role are precisely defined. Interaction within management tends to be vertical, i.e. between supervisor and subordinate. Operations and working behaviour are governed by instructions and decisions issued by superiors . . .'[17]

Where the 'environment' of the organisation was a rapidly changing one, an 'organic' system of management was more appropriate. In an 'organic system', 'jobs lose much of their formal definition in terms of methods, duties, and powers, which have to be redefined continually by interaction with others participating in a task. Interaction runs laterally as much as vertically. Communications between people of different ranks tend to resemble lateral consultation rather than vertical command. Omniscience can no longer be imputed to the head of the concern.'[18]

The work of Burns and Stalker is helpful because it suggests the circumstances in which some confusion over responsibilities may be a good thing. Where these circumstances exist an organic system of management will permit an easier adaptation to new tasks. In a mechanistic system of management there would be delays in responding to new demands because managers would wait until responsibility for them had been allocated by senior management. Delays, bottlenecks and harassed senior managers would be the consequence. Where responsibilities were usually ill-defined, at least at the boundary of a particular function, the new tasks would be more likely to be met more quickly by a manager taking them on. By way of elaboration it is worth underlining the consequence for formal relationships. Vertical relationships become less obviously hierarchal and lateral communication more important. Before we look at the relevance of this work for health service managers we need to make two further points. First, the descriptions of 'mechanistic' and 'organic' systems of managements are descriptions of polar types. An organisation can be more or less organic or mechanistic. Second, it may be that different parts of a large organisation like the health service, may demand different styles of management.

Is this theory of any relevance to the health service manager? Are the changes facing the health services of the same intensity and kind as those described in the studies of the electronics industry? Or are hospitals operating under the relatively stable conditions which make mechanistic systems appropriate? On balance we accept Spencer's view that where patients are involved, there will be much improvisation; the routine procedure is not wholly relevant.[19] At field level, then, the level of unpredictability is high which *prima facie* suggests the suitability of an organic system of management.

One of the most important front-line managers is the ward sister. She is the operational co-ordinator of the cure and care systems of the hospital. She acts as the representative of the doctor in clinical matters and obtains the necessary hotel services for her patients. In both capacities the quality of *lateral* relationships is crucial. She requires expertise as a service-seeker to communicate effectively with those departments who will deliver the correct records, the correct food, the correct laundry, the correct stores, the prescribed drugs, prescribed treatment and prescribed tests at the time she wants them.

In recent years both the hospital and local authority nursing services have been reorganised. The Salmon and Mayston systems of management are very similar and will be readily assimilable in the new service. Yet both systems emphasise responsibility up the line, a hierarchical system of relationships and communications upwards all of which Burns and Stalker suggested may be unhelpful where events were unpredictable. Significantly Williams has commented on the absence of lateral contacts in hospitals in South Wales.[20] Though his comments relate to a system of management which preceded Salmon, it is hard to see how this reform would have remedied this particular deficiency and indeed it may well have made things worse. If this is so it may explain why the new management structure for hospital nursing services is not seen as an unmixed blessing. So much so that by 1971 the *British Medical Journal* felt that so many doubts had been expressed about the utility of the Salmon structure that a halt should be called.[21]

More attention to lateral communications to allow relationships with other departmental heads to grow seems desirable. Yet this implies less supervision from above for the ward sister. This may have been achieved in the community health sector, where nurses have been attached to practices, and particularly when they are based in the surgery or health centre itself. Questions of priorities, and rationing of time have often to be settled between nurse and doctor without reference to any administrator in the local health authority. The popularity of these schemes with general practitioners is in marked contrast to many consultants' views of Salmon. No doubt the bilateral contact between the nurse and general practitioner which facilitates co-ordination through easier contact and greater understanding of the other's problems is a factor in this favourable response. The relationship between the district nurse and administrator where there are attachment schemes seems to be of a different texture to those in hospitals. The district nurse is more independent of her nursing superior. Nursing administrators in hospitals above ward level may have to accept a role more akin to that of an advisor, or perhaps a relationship nearer the staff/line manager model if lateral relationships are to grow and thus produce a system which is better able to cope with unpredictability and changing demand.

Again, there may be particular wards and departments, for example intensive care, active geriatric wards, etc., where the element of unpredictability is such that problems and requirements for action arise which cannot be broken down and distributed among specialist roles. On the other hand there are others where the environment is not changing rapidly and more mechanistic systems of management are appropriate. Medical records, laundry, finance and accounting (in spite of computerisation), supplies, stores and personnel may be examples of this type of department.

A health service manager will do well to look carefully at situations before deciding whether a more organic or mechanistic system of management is the most appropriate. He must be prepared, too, for considerable resistance from staff if he decides to move towards a more organic system. Where there is uncertainty many will seek security in more clearly defined duties, responsibilities and procedures. In the case of doctors, nurses and some front-line para-medical staff, this preference may in turn be reinforced by rigidly enforced codes to minimise the anxiety inherent in their work.[22] The insecurity arising both from this natural anxiety which close contact with patients evokes and a changing environment may explain why even before the Salmon reforms the nursing services in hospitals, for example, were a byword for mechanistic organisation. There were countless rules and clearly understood (if not always written) responsibilities and status hierarchies. The Salmon structure which defines responsibilities down to first-line management level and transfers some responsibility away from the ward, reinforces this process. And not only can it be criticised in terms of our argument that it introduces rigidity where flexibility is required in conditions of change. Menzies has argued that the systems that are created as defence mechanisms against anxiety may also serve to reduce job satisfaction.[23]

IV CO-ORDINATION WITHIN AUTHORITIES; CONCLUSION

The inadequate management system of the hospital service was held by many to be responsible for many of its shortcomings, particularly in the field of co-ordination. It provided another convenient line of defence, or alibi, for those who wished to avoid responsibility for the slow improvement in management performance.

We have suggested that expectations of the impact of reorganisation may be unrealistic as a result. Problems of co-ordination will still exist and indeed, given the pace of specialisation, intensify in the future. The success with which these problems are tackled will depend on the calibre of the manager. The calibre of the manager in turn will depend on a clear appreciation of the relevance of particular management theories to particular situations. There are no short cuts or panaceas.

9

The Constraints of Public Finance

I INTRODUCTION

We have now discussed two of the three ways in which the pre-reform structure of the health service was seen as unhelpful to the manager. We now turn to the third feature, the constraints of public finance, which gave rise to much criticism. Our focus is again the impact of these features of the organisation on the individual performance of managers. Were these features so important as to be a major obstacle to improved services? Or were they another convenient alibi?

It is of necessity a brief look. The financial arrangements for the new system are still not clear and that of the present hospital service is in the process of being changed. We must thus confine ourselves to general observations. Most of the comment concerns the financial system of the pre-reform hospital service since it approximates much more to what we can expect the new system to be, than does that of the local health authorities.

Ironically, Powell, in a comparison of the two, felt it was the local authority system that had more to commend it. Dependence on a local source of revenue produced a financial discipline and pride in existing services which was lacking in the hospital service.[1]

There were two types of financial controls which were seen as major obstacles to the manager trying to improve services:

(a) *Those arising from the method of budgetary control adopted for the hospital service*. In this category we include such constraints as the subjective form of accounting system adopted; the allocation of revenue on a historical basis; inability to carry over unspent balances; strict control over virement, etc. No doubt there were others which will be well known to readers but these were the most frequently cited ones.

(b) *Procedures to ensure there is no abuse of public funds*. In this category fall stores and inventory controls, procedures governing

70

allocation and control of patients' moneys, certification of claims for overtime, car journeys on official business, etc.

II OBSTACLES ARISING FROM THE FORM OF BUDGETARY CONTROL

There is little doubt that the subjective method of budgeting (and for that matter most of the statistics) did not produce the most appropriate information for hospital staff who were trying to maximise the use of resources. This is a criticism which has been made many times and need not be laboured here. There have been many attempts to produce more useful information to managers (costing schemes, hospital activity analysis, etc.) but these, too, have come under fire.

The alternatives to the present system are not self-evident. Certainly there are some alternatives in the wings which have their champions (e.g. planned programme budgeting). At the time of writing a change-over to departmental budgeting is under way. But all fall foul of the same obstacle – the absence of clear-cut objectives and norms. Montacute has pointed out in relation to budgetary allocations how valuable it would be 'if standards could be established to indicate what is a reasonable level of service and what is a reasonable cost'.[2] This information is not so far forthcoming.

This same problem also makes the production of more useful statistics difficult. Unless one is quite sure what it is which needs to be measured and that the criteria used actually do measure what it purports to do, the usefulness of management information is clearly impaired.

There would, however, be agreement that the information produced now is of increasing help to the *determined* and *resourceful* managers who are clear about *their* operational objectives. Much, too, depends on the treasurer. The many examples of helpful information provided by treasurers illustrate again that this organisational constraint is an obstacle which some manage to surmount. From experience, this, too, would seem to be true of the alleged difficulties surrounding *virement*. Resourceful heads of departments and group secretaries have found this obstacle much more easily surmountable than some would have us believe. The real criticism of present financial and management information is that they provide a convenient refuge for the less resourceful and determined.

Unspent balances, or rather the stories of rash spending in the month before the end of the financial year, threaten to become the folklore and myths of the unreformed national health service.[3] The much more important objection, however, to the central system of financing of which this criticism is but a part, is the lack of financial incentive to be efficient. 'Mr C. A. Montacute suggested that in the hospital service it did not pay to be efficient or critical. There was no incentive . . .'[4] Without such an incentive, efforts to find the extra resources from existing allocations were less thorough than they might have been. Yet there is no obvious alternative. And a budgetary system which provided incentives to managers to be efficient would create some difficult problems. Should the 'savings' resulting from increased efficiency within a department be transferred to other departments or other districts which may need extra resources because they have not been so diligent? If the head of department has managed to cut his budget by two per cent without reducing quality, should he lose that two per cent next year? If not, why should he reduce the two per cent? They may be familiar questions but so far there are no familiar answers. Until answers are found, Montacute's criticisms of the 'old' system and probably any new way of financing the health services are valid. They are also extensions of Powell's criticisms of the effect of central financing on local managerial responsibility.

How can we build in acceptable incentives to be efficient? There will be a different system of accounting and budgetary control in the new service. Yet it is unlikely to provide the incentive to be efficient. We must rely again on the managerial skills of the personnel in the service. The answer lies in their motivation as much as structural reform. The pre-reform structure did not *totally* block or stifle these motivations. Otherwise, how does one explain the behaviour of those managers whose efficiency was high?

III   PROCEDURES TO ENSURE PROPRIETY OF EXPENDITURE

This is the other type of constraint imposed by the fact of public finance. The existence of auditors reminds managers of the importance of correct as well as efficient expenditure. Public finance is assumed to demand higher levels of propriety than in the private sector. This is often said to be another reason why managers are often hindered in their attempts to cut costs to free funds for development elsewhere.

In the planning of a new hospital in which the author was involved this dilemma presented itself very clearly over the type of telephone exchange which should be installed. The dilemma centred on the means of making external calls. Subscriber trunk dialling had recently been introduced. Should external calls be mainly or almost totally through an operator? Or should extensions have the facility to dial external calls? If individuals' extensions had direct access to outside lines, would there be considerable abuse? Would personal calls be made without appropriate payment? The cost of these would be difficult to control. Yet the obvious means of controlling this abuse – all outside calls through the telephone operator – would probably mean considerably higher expenditure. Another consideration in the days of high employment was the unavailability of suitable staff. Extensions with direct access to lines outside the hospital would require fewer operators, thus directly reducing the cost of operating an exchange and finding suitable staff. The project team came down on the side of efficiency with the proviso that there should be controls over the number of extensions from which external calls could be dialled directly.

This dilemma has been faced nationally on the question of linen in hospitals. Less counting of linen means a greater loss. Yet frequent counting by ward and departmental staff is expensive in time, energy and tempers. The decision to discontinue elaborate checks at ward level was a triumph for the criterion of efficiency over correctness.

Elsewhere perhaps the requirements of propriety are more strongly upheld. To the extent this is so the criterion of propriety is a constraint on improved performance. But to the extent this is allowed to be so is also dependent to some degree on managers in the service. There is sufficient discretion locally to ensure that too great a priority is not given to propriety where this clashes with efficiency. And for those who feel that the dictates of efficiency should be paramount, there *is* support from '*them*'. 'A prime objective of financial control is to ensure that value is obtained for expenditure incurred.'[5]

It is clear that an undue emphasis on propriety is another convenient rock for those who prefer the security of blaming 'them' for the lack of additional funds for development.

IV CONCLUSION

A major theme in the reform of the service is managerial efficiency.

If this intention is translated into practice, it may lessen the emphasis on 'correctness' of expenditure where this is at the expense of efficiency.

Clearly there are limits to this process. Where public money is being expended there will be quite proper demands for elaborate safeguards. There is also another limiting factor. Some of the financial information and statistics will still be required in forms other than those necessitated by the criterion of efficiency. The representatives of the community will require from the government of the day and the Department information which they can appreciate and think important. Their appreciative systems and estimate of what is important (e.g. the renal dialysis issue) will differ in some respects from those responsible for providing the services. This can be an important corrective if the objectives of the providers are out of harmony with those of the consumer (e.g. in the provision of facilities for geriatric patients). Increasingly in the future these considerations will not determine the form of all statistics and financial information. There will be opportunities for managers to break out a little more from the dictates of propriety rather than efficiency. Whether these opportunities are grasped will depend on the manager, as it has done in the past. The organisational constraints are only as big an obstacle as he wants to make them.

10

What can the Managers in the Health Service Manage?

I INTRODUCTION

The main theme of the book is how to improve the service. We have argued that the popular prescriptions – more money, more staff, better hospitals, and unified control over health services – are either unrealistic or will have a smaller impact than some expect. Indeed one problem of the reform of the National Health Service may be the unrealistic expectations of its effect held by some in the service.[1] The most effective way to improve services is a more efficient use of *present* resources, and this in turn depends on better management. This is more likely if unrealistic expectations are scaled down and less energy is devoted to finding scapegoats. 'Being fallible, most of us find substandards easier to attain than standards and are ever ready to invent constraints outside ourselves, even where none exist. Efficiency can be frightening.'[2]

We are now ready to look more closely at the contribution which those in the service can make to improving it. What can individual members or departments hope to achieve? Or put rather differently, what standards can reasonably be expected of them? Once these questions are answered we can be clearer about the degree to which we can then hold those who provide the service responsible for inadequate development of it.

We begin by discussing some general reactions which the author has had to the thesis that much of the responsibility for initiating and engineering improvements lies with those who run the service. This is followed by an analysis of the influence which staff in the service seem to wield now. In the next chapter we look at the sources of this influence as a prelude to establishing the degree of responsibility of those running the service to improve it.

Responsibility for increasing efficiency and innovation, and ideally commensurate accountability, is not of course shared equally. Some staff are more powerful than others. This obvious

75

fact of organisational life is another alibi for staff who wish to divert attention from their own responsibilities. 'Don't talk to us about improving our services, you must talk to our bosses,' is one typical response. These 'bosses' for middle managers from the hospital service have turned out to be senior group officers, who in the perception of the course members are the controllers of resources. Particular sticking points in the organisation which receive frequent mention have been group secretaries, treasurers, supplies officers, matrons, chief nursing officers, group engineers and consultants. These and other comments are frequently substantiated with explanations. 'I'm always making suggestions but *they* never listen' or 'we ask for things, but are never told what *their* decision is'.

What is interesting is that on one occasion in which the author participated in a first-line management course the same comments were made. The only difference was that the level at which suggestions 'stuck', and where response was unhelpful had changed. It was now fixed at the level of the middle managers. In the higher reaches of the organisation the same phenomenon is found. Senior group officers make similar comments of regional staff ('failed doctors', 'never been in a hospital') and regional hospital board staff of Department staff (what do *they* know about running a hospital service?).

Similar comments, though less frequently, have been made to the author in a somewhat briefer acquaintance with community health service personnel. 'It's the doctor whose holding up our attachment schemes . . .' No doubt the same phenomena is found in executive council services.

If these comments are to be taken at face value the calibre of successive tiers of health service organisation must diminish as one nears the apex. Even if there is some truth in the Peter Pringle argument that one is promoted to the point above one's level of competence, this is asking a little too much of the observer to accept. However, these reactions do underline some important features of organisational life which are important to any assessment of the influence of staff in the service.

First, it demonstrates the junior's perceptions of his boss. This is important for motivating staff. Second, it demonstrates in a simplistic way the difficulties of evaluating who is responsible for what in a complex organisation. And that it is even more difficult in an organisation which employs so many professional staff. Third, it also demonstrates again the importance of scapegoats and alibis. Could it be that work in the health service provokes so much anxiety that there is a preference for non-responsibility? Or at best accepting only a very diffuse responsibility? Some feel this may be particularly true of organisations in which a large proportion of staff are women.[3] Women, particularly married ones, may prefer less responsibility rather than more because it fits their traditional position more closely and because of the family demands made on them.

There is evidence that staff involved in the day-to-day running of welfare services do have more influence on events than these disclaimers would suggest.

'They are not simply the instruments of the governing body – an impersonal link between the committee and its clients. They create, and continually modify, the services. . . . Those providing the service are concerned with the improvement and development of their work within the limits determined by available power and resources, and according to the aspirations derived from their colleagues, their training, their professional loyalties and personal needs.'[4]

This was one assessment of the contribution of social and welfare workers to the development of their services. It was an assessment based on a number of administrative case studies most of which involved British social services.

Do and can providers in the health service create, and continually modify, the service . . .? Or are they more restricted than providers in other social welfare organisations? Some may argue that it is so, at least for hospitals:

'Why then are hospitals a byword for authoritarianism? The hierarchical character of hospital medical and nursing organisation is notorious. Status differences are almost as marked among the non-professional as among the professional groups, supervisors expect strict obedience from subordinates: and hospitals probably have more rules and regulations than most organisations.'[5]

The explanation for this state of affairs is intolerance of error and ambiguity where human life is often at stake. When Spencer acknowledges, however, the need for collaboration for events for which there is no appropriate regulation he is acknowledging the need for initiative beyond formal requirements. He expects *more* from individuals than is routinely prescribed. Even if we accept the accuracy of Spencer's description, there *is* scope for initiative. If he has over-estimated the mechanistic character of hospitals it follows there is even more room for initiative. The exact nature of hospital organisation, as are the views on what it ought to be, is still a matter of dispute. But this is a subject we can leave to others. All we need to establish here is that even in a mechanistic system as described by Spencer those providing the service have room for manoeuvre.

These are general assertions. We need to be more specific about which health service staff have this influence on events and the extent of the room for manoeuvre. We can reach a considered judgement on both these points by looking at their power to obstruct change before turning to their contribution to innovation.

II   THE POWER TO OBSTRUCT

Change initiated and approved by the controllers of resources requires the support and acquiescence of middle and first-line managers if it is to be successfully implemented. Non-implementation or distortion of policy by middle-ranking and junior staff is not unknown. Spencer feels this to be a lesser but not a non-existent risk in hospitals because 'the goals of individual members and the objectives of the organisation are much more likely to coincide than they do in other organisations.'[6] No doubt he would feel this to be true of the community health services too. But this observation does not deny the power of providers; it stresses rather the infrequency with which it is used.

Children in hospital

However, there are many examples of how official objectives have either been ignored or distorted. The example of the children's ward sister who kept parents waiting until the recommended hours for visiting children is one.[7] Gerda Cohen describes a similar experience: ' "We did away with restrictions ages ago," said one matron, weightily propelling me past a large notice: Visiting from 4.30 to 5.0 p.m. daily. Identical placards hung outside all the wards. "We keep them up", Matron smiled at my naive mystification "because otherwise visitors would think they could pop in any time." '[8] Both examples post-date the Platt Report on the welfare of children in hospital which gave professional blessing to the ending of restrictions on visiting, and which the Ministry of Health commended to hospital authorities. The first example post-dates the start of Robertson's campaign to waken hospitals to the dangers of maternal deprivation by fifteen years! And even in 1972 the Department of Health again thought it necessary to have to repeat its advice on the importance of contact between parents and child.[9] Clearly the official position on the visiting of children, particularly by parents, did not guarantee what would happen in practice. And senior management had not sufficient authority to ensure that their policy was carried out to the letter by those providing the service.

Another personal experience illustrates the influence of the provider on how policy is implemented. The writer's own eighteen-month-old child was admitted for observation late in the evening to a paediatric ward in a new hospital. He was obviously terrified, and resisted attempts by staff to examine him. His screams during examination were clearly heard in the nearby waiting area where his parents sat. When the doctor returned, she was told that his mother would like to stay the night since there was insufficient time to settle the child and get home the same evening. Domestic arrangements were satisfactory; the father and grandparents could look after the other children. There was a slight hesitation before the Registrar said that they preferred the parents' overnight accommodation, which was unoccupied, to be kept for parents of very ill children. There was another pause – would the parents withdraw their request? The pressures to do so were strong. The doctor made it clear she thought a maternal presence was unnecessary. In the end it was the combined strength of the parents (and knowledge of departmental policy) which managed to resist this moral pressure. They chose to insist, provided the room was not being used for the parent of a very sick child.

The rights and wrongs of the issue are irrelevant to this discussion. What is relevant is the influence of the doctor even when senior management has specified the rules. The 'spirit' of the departmental advice is obvious: but what happens on the ground may differ because of the power of those who provide the service to 'adjust' policy.

Scandals in long-stay hospitals

More serious examples of the power of staff are the various 'scandals' in long-stay hospitals. The variation in standards both between and within the same hospitals demonstrates the 'power' of the charge nurse and ward sister. Given identical environmental conditions (ward layout, equipment, staff) some charge nurses condoned or participated in unnecessary brutality while others did not. A glimpse of their power was given by the Committee of Inquiry on Farleigh Hospital.

'The nursing staff fell into two groups: a tightly-knit group of trained staff and their families, firmly in control at ward level . . . and a group of student nurses, state enrolled nurses, nursing assistants, ward orderlies and others, who, as relative newcomers, inexperienced and less conforming were more critical of the conditions they found. We were told by members of the second group that they were laughed at by ward staff when they complained: that senior staff ignored their complaints because they had no corroborative evidence . . .'[10]

It will be argued that such situations are untypical. This may be so, though perhaps the frequency of the scandals in the late 1960s and early 1970s ought to temper this view. Even if the *cruelty* is untypical then conditions which give so much power to the providers is not so rare. In long-stay hospitals, with comparatively few medical staff, the power of the nursing staff may be proportionately greater than that of their counterparts in acute hospitals. But it demonstrates, even if such hospitals are not typical of all hospitals, the power of the providers to ignore, bend and in a few cases openly flout rules.

The case of the missing bottles of milk
Thirty bottles of milk were delivered daily to a paediatric ward of twenty-four children. For various reasons (economy, control of expenditure and an alternative to cereals in cold weather) the catering officer decided that he would send six fewer bottles of milk to the ward and use it for porridge. This, of course, would provide the equivalent nutrition (at least potentially) for patients. Communications were rather faulty and the ward sister objected strongly to the decision. Explanations and arguments did not change her mind.

One of her complaints was that the porridge was cold when it reached the ward. Attempts were made to check the accuracy of the complaints. Eventually, according to the catering officer, there was a particularly long delay on the ward before the porridge was served. The hospital secretary had the container of cold porridge put on his desk so that he could vouch for its coldness! In the subsequent confrontation the sister was asked to account for her use of the thirty pints of milk which she could not do. The catering officer suspected (as they all do!) that some of the unaccounted-for milk found its way into staff beverages!

The outcome was interesting. The missing bottles of milk were restored and the ward sister agreed to prepare instant porridge herself.

This is a description of the issue from the viewpoint of the catering officer: it may be partial. However, the means available to one departmental head (the sister) to exert pressure on another (catering officer) are clear. She can demonstrate the inadequacy of the service he is offering and by which he will be partially judged by his seniors. In this case it was successfully done.

The three examples highlight the power of some managers in some hospitals. It is unlikely that their peers in other hospitals are less influential. What of staff in the community health services?

Attachment of district nurses and health visitors to particular general practitioners may well have helped to make community nurses even more independent than their peers in hospitals. Decisions on priorities are now more likely to be settled by joint decisions of the nurse and general practitioner. Previously an administrative nurse would in most cases have been involved. One director of nursing services talking about the changeover to attachment schemes in her area said this byproduct of reform had created some anxieties among front-line staff. The nurses had been uneasy at being handed these responsibilities.

The three examples illustrate different facets of the power to obstruct. The first two demonstrated clearly that the ward sisters had power not only to influence policy passed down from above, but to hinder efforts by their peers (or their seniors) to introduce changes which they considered detrimental. In the cases of visiting on paediatric wards and brutality in some long-stay wards, the front-line staff chose to turn a blind eye to some instructions coming to them from the same vertical channels of command. The relationship between first-line and senior staff owed something to the use to which the first-line providers wanted to put them, as well as the formal descriptions of what it should be.

The third illustration highlights the importance of the contribution of those who run the service to the texture of lateral relationships. Relationships with other departmental staff are not always amenable to commands from above. The commandment to 'love thy neighbour' operates only in limited contexts.

These are examples of the more negative aspects of the power of the providers. The merits of the issues are only of passing interest. They serve to illustrate the basic point we are making. Middle and first-line managers have power, and their support for change is crucial to its successful implementation. In less structured situations than hospitals that power will be correspondingly greater. But this leaves open the question of whether they have the opportunity for the more positive role that Donnison and Chapman described for other social welfare workers. What opportunities have they to innovate? or to ensure themselves a decisive voice in the counsels of senior management?

III   THE POWER TO INNOVATE

There is no ready answer to these questions. Much more research is required to test the validity of Donnison and Chapman's hypotheses when applied to the health service. Others may reasonably object that local situations vary greatly. In some areas staff may have such power, but this does not mean it is generally true. It may also be true that the boundaries beyond which they cannot go may be more tightly drawn in some areas than in others. Yet there are sufficient examples of innovation in which local managers are often the moving spirit to suggest that the hypotheses about their actual or potential role in the health service is not entirely inappropriate.

Postgraduate Medical Education Centres
One of the most spectacular and rapid developments in the health service has been the growth of postgraduate medical education centres. In the early 1960s there were few such centres. In 1969 there were over eighty in England and Wales alone. Few would doubt their success or popularity among medical staff. But who decided that such centres should develop? Sir George Godber's assessment is as follows.

'I cannot overemphasise the importance of the spontaneous nature of this development within the profession itself. It did not arise from the prompting of the central department, however much it may have been assisted from central funds. The Nuffield Provincial Hospitals Trust and Sir George Pickering, Chairman of its Medical Committee, picked up the initiative of two medical groups in Exeter and Stoke on Trent and helped it to become the general movement it now is.'[11]

An Emergency Chemical Pathology Service in Central London[12]
One of the major problems facing laboratories are emergency requests for services outside normal working hours. In the case of chemical pathology tests these problems are accentuated by the fall in the quality of work done outside normal working hours. This is partly due to the fact that pathologists and technicians may be called upon to do tests for which they are not trained or experienced.

To try and overcome these problems, fourteen London hospitals, with a total of 4,500 beds, collaborated in 1971 to provide a centralised emergency service based on one laboratory. The emergency service is manned by eight medical students who already hold an honours degree in biochemistry or chemistry.

The system of regular duties by the graduates who work one full night and one evening out of eight solves some of the difficulties arising from 'on call' systems. Also as students they are highly motivated and thus provide a source of staff of a high calibre. Considerable advantages have resulted. 'The major advantage is accuracy, attributable to the initial intensive training and general proficiency of the students, the availability of modern equipment, and the use of adequate numbers of standards and quality control sera.' More demands are being made on the service as confidence grows and the cost per test is being reduced.[13]

There is no reference in the article to the originator or originators of the idea. There is no reference either to the member of staff (if he was a different person) who took up the idea and piloted it through the necessary procedures. The acknowledgment of the 'help and encouragement' of hospital administrative and some Departmental staff does suggest that much of the initiative came from the providers of the service themselves.

Interim comment

There are three objections to the use of these examples to demonstrate the contribution of providers to innovation in the health service. The first is the one mentioned above. There have been no organisational studies of the health services of the calibre of those by Donnison and Chapman, and thus we cannot say that an underlying organisational situation which allowed local managers to take initiatives is a normal one. All we can say is that both Sir George Godber and the authors of the article on the emergency chemical pathology service do see scope for the 'providers' to innovate. And both are radical innovations, with wider implications.

A second objection relates to the occupation of the staff in question. It is probably much easier for medical staff to innovate and get their suggestions accepted because there are fewer bureaucratic constraints placed upon them than other groups of staff in the service. Hence, it may be true that changes do come about as a result of efforts of some personnel in the service but this is not true of them all. Clearly, we cannot expect the laboratory technician, the pharmacist, the radiographer or the ward sister to be as influential or powerful as the doctor. In addition there is the obvious point that, in the field of treatment, doctors can adopt new techniques or try new ones with little or no interference from anyone else. Even when additional resources are required and have to be solicited then their exalted position makes it much easier for them to obtain those resources than it would have been for lesser mortals.

Yet factors other than status and its correlate bargaining power must enter into the decision of controllers to offer the 'help and encouragement' necessary for success. In both examples, the controllers' support had to be gained before the project could get off the ground successfully. Though others may find it more difficult to obtain that 'help and encouragement', it can be and is obtained in many cases. The possibility and indeed the probability is there. The example of medical staff taking a leading role in innovation illustrates the mechanisms within organisations by which change is sometimes introduced. We can legitimately expect similar things from non-medical staff.

Third, in both cases, the initiatives led to a successful claim for *additional* resources. We have argued that the major problem for the health service is to motivate staff to use *existing* resources more efficiently in order to produce the 'surplus' for new developments. Thus the two illustrations were inappropriate. However, the choice of examples can be defended by pointing to the probable unquantifiable savings the changes produced elsewhere. In the case of the emergency chemical pathology service quicker diagnosis should lead to speedier discharge, and fewer delays because of the reduction in the number of errors in reporting would produce savings in staff time. However, such a defence for our choice is unnecessary at this stage. The examples have been chosen to demonstrate the power and influence of those who provide the service to innovate. Evidence on the contribution of other professional groups and middle- and first-line managers to innovation *is* scarcer. Examples, if the nursing press is typical, are fewer. This is not evidence that nurses do not influence change. It is as easily explained by their different interests, and their judgement on what issues are worth writing up. However, there are examples known to the writer of initiatives taken by non-medical providers.

The disappearing physiotherapy service
The power of the non-medical provider to take the initiative (though the end result was the reverse of development!) was

amply demonstrated by the success with which one Superintendent Physiotherapist in the north of England reduced the services offered by his department.

The physiotherapy services in a large acute hospital were increasingly restricted in 1971. The Superintendent explained that the shortage of suitably trained physiotherapy staff made this necessary. The local newspaper frequently reported cases of patients who needed physiotherapy but were unable to obtain it or for whom treatment would stop prematurely.

In a situation of this type, if the controllers or determiners of demand wished to try and maintain the status quo, the 'power' of the Superintendent is sufficient to ensure that such a view could hardly prevail. In the final analysis only the physiotherapist can judge what standard of service can be provided with a certain number of staff. It may be – hypothetically – that other staff could press for priority consideration more strongly than they could, for example, against a consultant who felt it necessary to restrict his services. Even if this is so, the basic point remains valid. The physiotherapist's agreement is essential and his or her judgement of what can be done must be largely accepted, though no doubt the formal approval of senior management would be required.

Nurses and innovation

There are examples in the nursing press of the contribution of nurses to innovation, but these are usually of a more pragmatic type. For example, there is a report of a matron of a hospital in Gloucester, who with the health visitor and a designer, produced a prototype of a do-it-yourself pram for patients suffering from congenital dislocation of the hip.[14] At ward level Dr Baker's 1971 report on the hospital advisory service mentions the importance of encouraging initiative as

'significant improvements usually follow. For example, on one ward for elderly patients the ward nurses had developed their own routine and some patients were given breakfast in bed in rotation, followed by a period when they had extra attention and considerable efforts were made to improve the appearance of each. On admission wards, nurses can create small groups, each with its own identity and relationship with a particular nurse.'[15]

Clearly some nurses obviously had the power to initiate changes in routine and used it to best advantage.

However, nurses do not have to wait until they are 'allowed' to use their initiative. Like the physiotherapist, they have sufficient power in some areas of nursing service to give senior management little option but to do what they want. Two fuller illustrations will perhaps make this process clearer.

The case of theatre changing rooms

In this case there was one theatre changing room for a staff of three men and sixteen women. The complications that arose, even in 1972, can be easily envisaged. There was 'sympathy and understanding' from the matron and the hospital secretary, and a second changing room was promised for the financial year 1969/70. It was not provided and after again being promised in 1970/1 it still did not materialise.

At this point the Superintendent acted. The three lockers for the male employees were put out in the corridor where they were now expected to change. The second theatre changing room was then provided as a priority item.

The case of the upgraded men's wards

This is an illustration taken from an article in the nursing press written by a regional officer. [16] The perspective from which the events are viewed is somewhat different from the one in the previous illustrations. On this occasion it is written from the perspective of a senior manager who discusses the efforts of a charge nurse.

The ward contained eighty-two severely disturbed and handicapped men. At a time when the regional board was obviously taking an interest in upgrading two large wards with an ablutions block, 'he was challenged to move his unruly band from the bare necessities of living into a home from home'. His main problem 'lay with the staffing level'. He got the importance and scale of this problem over to the controllers 'by measuring the gap and the effects of closing it, and then organising a practical demonstration to support his findings'. The principal regional nursing officer acknowledged that 'the resulting evidence, to his great credit, was overwhelmingly persuasive'.

In the case of the theatre changing rooms senior management was virtually compelled to act by the decision of the theatre superintendent to make the male staff change in the corridor. The decision about the priority of the changing room was to a large extent pre-empted by the superintendent. In the second case the channels through which pressure was exerted were more orthodox ones. But having given encouragement, the regional officers would have found it more difficult to say 'no' in face of the effective way the charge nurse took his opportunity to present his case. In both cases they had little option but to agree with the providers of the service.

Visiting grandfather

Those who give formal approval are not necessarily the most decisive element in any decision. One charge nurse who once tried to convince fellow students on a management course that it was, inadvertently undermined his own case.

He told of an incident when a mother asked whether her children could visit her ailing father. The rule was quite clear: no visiting by children. The charge nurse responded to the request by explaining the rule and saying it was not his responsibility. However, he advised the mother to go and see the hospital secretary as he was the representative of the management committee who made the rules. The charge nurse also told her to inform the secretary that it was 'all right' by him if the children visited their grandfather.

The charge nurse quoted this incident as evidence that he had no power in the matter: all power resided in the secretary. But his own description of what happened belies this. The charge nurse takes two decisions. First, to send the mother to the secretary who is then 'put on the spot'. Second, to give the mother's request his blessing. It is hard to see how the secretary in such a situation could have refused the request. To do so would have involved him publicly going against the charge nurse's judgement and making a decision without the knowledge, expertise and perhaps help of the charge nurse.

This argument obviously cannot be taken too far. In certain areas of policy the contribution of senior management is decisive. But at the level of service at which we are talking there is considerable scope for initiative for professional and other managerial staff. There is sufficient scope, too, to bring about changes and attract additional resources.

IV CONCLUSION – WHAT CAN THE PROVIDERS DO?

Our analysis of the power of staff who manage the service started with disclaimers to any real influence. It is obvious from the illustrations that *some* have more power in some areas of practice than these disclaimers would lead us to believe. It may be true that medical staff, pharmacists, and engineers have more power in attracting resources, introducing changes and in obstructing change of which they disapprove than others, for example, nurses. This observation receives support from Julia Davies' assessment of first-line management courses for ward sisters in the Manchester region.[17] She points out that nurses do find it difficult to act as 'change agents' when they return to hospitals. A more considered judgement on the applicability of Donnison and Chapman's hypothesis about nursing staff who 'create and continually modify the service' must clearly await more evidence. However, the hypothesis is not disproved in the health service since it is clearly possible for some to behave in this way.

The disclaimers are at least partly explained by traditional notions of the proper functions of middle and first-line management. Top management is acknowledged to be the innovator and the policy-maker and the lower ranks are mere executives. The theories which understate the power of some middle- and first-line managers to obstruct, modify and innovate may have to be developed or disregarded. The facts of the situation are probably quite different. What we may be witnessing is a cultural lag whereby common perceptions based on these traditional theories are taking longer to modify.

11

The Contribution of Health Service Managers

There are two important corollaries of the thesis that the power of those managing the service is greater than formal descriptions suggest. First, how can we maximise that contribution? The answer to this question may lie in a clearer appreciation of the sources of their power. A better understanding is a prerequisite to a more effective deployment of influence. Second, power involves responsibility. The responsibility of staff for innovation should be more explicitly acknowledged if this thesis is accepted. Can we not, for example, hold those who provide the service responsible (in some degree) for lack of development?

I SOURCES OF POWER

So far we have not specified very precisely what we mean by power and influence. In the subsequent discussion we follow Mechanic and define power as 'any force that results in behaviour that would not have occurred if the force had not been present'.[1]

Clearly, power is affected by the degree of dependence on others. Dependence on those who provide the service owes much to their guardianship of a body of professional knowledge. Neither the controller of resources nor other staff can prescribe action within the area acknowledged to be 'professional'. They depend on the professional for information (e.g. on the practicality of new procedures) and the application of that particular body of knowledge. The area of professional discretion is a large one, particularly where prestigious occupations are involved. The larger the area the more dependent are fellow employees.

The full extent of this professional territory and the dependence of others can be seen in decisions on which patient, or patient group, is given priority of access, particularly to specialised treatment.

'One of the problems, therefore, within a fully developed health service, may be the ordering of priorities in accordance with a dispassionate assessment of the benefit to the community served. Paradoxically it may even be necessary to ensure that services such as pathological or radiological investigations are not undertaken without full justification. This may sound a cold-blooded exercise in logistics and that is just what it would be if a central department tried to lay down priorities: it is surely vital in societies such as ours that decisions shall be made on medical grounds by the doctors themselves . . .'[2]

This is not to say the consultant is 'autonomous'. The area of decision-making where he exercises his untrammelled professional judgement is on one side bounded by those decisions where the collective judgement of medical staff is required: Sir George Godber suggested some decisions on priorities may fall into this category. It is bounded on another side by his own lack of expertise in certain fields and therefore dependence on others (e.g. chemical pathology, pharmacology). It is again bounded by the need to persuade others where additional resources are required (e.g. additional nurses or equipment). But within his sphere he is virtually autonomous because he controls access to information. He knows: others do not. But where he has not got the information he is dependent on others, just as he is on those who control access to resources.

Not all professionals are in such a strong position as the medical profession. Nurses, physiotherapists, social workers, health visitors and others find their acknowledged sphere of competence narrower and their advice correspondingly more likely to be unsolicited or ignored. People are less dependent on them because they control access to either a less valuable or less extensive field of expertise. Etzioni has suggested we should classify such groups differently. He suggests the label 'semi-professionals'.[3] These are groups of workers with a distinctive organisational role in that they have more autonomy than, say, clerical staff but, unlike doctors, usually work in a hierarchical setting. Their supervisors are usually fellow semi-professionals. Although their guardianship of a theoretical body of knowledge is less acknowledged, they have expertise and information which creates considerable dependence on them. A scheme for upgrading a department could not proceed satisfactorily without the help and perhaps consent of the head of the department, be it a kitchen, health centre, ante-natal clinic, ward, physiotherapy or radiography department. The administrator, engineer and building supervisor would need the information at the disposal of the semi-professional. It is true that the position of doctors gives them the right to be consulted (and veto) on a wider range of matters than the semi-professional. But this is a matter of degree, and other members of the organisation are dependent on the information and expertise of semi-professionals. It is their access to this specialised information which gives them so much say in organisations.

Another illustration of the importance of access to a body of knowledge is demonstrated by the changing relationship between the established and newly qualified professional. A newly qualified member of staff is often more authoritative because he has been exposed to the new techniques and information that have materialised since the older staff qualified. And this is exacerbated where established staff are increasingly engaged in administration which reduces opportunity to keep up to date with technical developments. In some respects the newer staff are more authoritative and control access to information which their seniors require. Seniors can be dependent on junior staff who in turn may have correspondingly more power than their predecessors in an age when the pace of discovery was less hectic. An inability to recognise this changing relationship between the newly qualified and the elder statesman can produce inappropriate management structures.

Another reason for the strong position of the professional is the mode of practice of some of them. The nurse, the therapist, the medical social worker, the health visitor and the radiographer are regularly in a face-to-face relationship with the patient. This contact is usually unsupervised, regulated only by professional norms. Others are clearly dependent on the professional competence of the member of staff and the information gained in these encounters. In particular, the doctor is very dependent on information gained by nurses and other para-medical staff in such face-to-face contacts. Refusal to pass on information is a useful way of bringing the houseman down a peg or two.

Guardianship of a body of knowledge (and therefore power) has so far been described as a 'professional' phenomenon. There is also information available to 'lower participants'[4] in organisations which is not a professional preserve, but which senior management requires. This is a source of power, together with a control of access to certain instrumentalities and persons which strengthens the position of the operational staff *vis-à-vis* senior management.

One of these factors is length of tenure. A long-serving employee who 'knows the ropes' has information vital to the newcomer. It is this factor which is acknowledged to diminish the impact which, for example, a new secretary of state might have on the health service. A permanent employee is in a particularly good position to point out the problems which might beset any change. His co-operation, too, in directing the minister to the key persons in the organisation is invaluable.

This is also an important factor in nursing. A large number of state-registered nurses never wander far from their training hospital.[5] They become in time the pillars of the local service, intuitively aware of their power through long working knowledge of the organisation. It is no surprise that new senior nurses sometimes find it difficult to get changes, for example on the visiting of children, implemented by them.

Another organisational factor which enhances the power of the lower participants is the strategic position some of them occupy in the communications system. An obvious example is the personal secretary. She guards access to her boss: she passes on requests and messages. The tone, or the promptness, or the accuracy with which these requests and messages are transmitted, are obviously important. Since she channels many of them, her power often seems so much greater than her formal position (or salary!) would warrant! Another key position is that of ward sister. She is the link between the cure and care systems of the hospital. As co-ordinator she requests or supervises the services offered. There is a wealth of information available at this point and doctors, in particular, are very dependent on the ward sister's production of it in the right form and at the right time. The unequal relationship between ward sisters and junior medical staff (ward sisters are often *de facto* in command) owes as much to this factor as it does to her longer service in the particular ward or department. She knows the rules and procedures of the hospital better than the doctor; she can make him look foolish by not offering information or being particularly diligent about doing what he suggests. In this way the junior doctor in particular becomes dependent on the ward sister both for information and access to services.

Mechanic argues this dependence is even more pronounced where the doctor acknowledges the impossibility of doing everything and delegates some of his responsibilities to the nurse. He quotes research which pointed to the

'implicit trading agreement (which) developed between physicians and attendants whereby attendants would take on some of the responsibilities and obligations of the ward physician in return for increased power in decision-making processes concerning patients. Failure of the ward physician to honour his part of the agreement resulted in the information being withheld, disobedience, lack of co-operation, and unwillingness of the attendants to serve as a barrier between the physician and a ward full of patients demanding attention and recognition. When the attendant withheld co-operation, the physician had difficulty in making a graceful entrance and departure from the ward, in handling necessary paperwork (officially his responsibility) and in obtaining information needed to deal adequately with daily treatment and behaviour problems. When attendants opposed change, they could wield influence by refusing to assume responsibilities officially assigned to the physician.'[6]

Those who argue that such a state of affairs is unlikely to exist in Britain are referred to the Farleigh inquiry.

'. . . In the case of patients prone to outbursts of violence the nursing staff had discretion to administer extra drugs, within the limits he (the psychiatrist) prescribed. On his visits to Farleigh he would see only those patients brought forward by the nursing staff and those detained patients whose status was under review . . .'[7]

The description of the delegation of medical responsibilities fits that of Mechanic's perfectly, although the committee of enquiry may have seen the causation a little differently. The psychiatrist becomes heavily dependent on nursing staff and they in turn have considerable opportunities to embarrass him (e.g. by working to rule!) if he wishes to change the relationship.

Another factor making lower participants guardians of gateways to information includes the interests of the senior managers. Their interest in 'major policy' (whatever this means!) and planning inevitably precludes close involvement in the mundane tasks of running the service. The independence of the lower participants is commensurately increased. The example of visiting children illustrates this process well. The subject was not a major interest of administrators in the 1950s and 1960s. What happened on the wards, within limits, was up to the ward sister. Consequently, information on what actually happened was the exclusive property of the sister. The administrator was dependent on her analysis of what was required and happening. Only when an alternative source of information (to that provided by the nurse and paediatrician) became available to the administrator (official publications from pressure groups) and there was some public pressure was there more attention paid to the problem.

It is the combination of guardianship of knowledge and expertise, together with organisational factors which strengthen the position of lower participants, which gives the professionals in the service more influence than their formal position suggests.

II   THE CREATIVE USE OF THE INFLUENCE AND POWER OF THOSE WHO PROVIDE THE SERVICE

While Mechanic and other writers have emphasised the contribution of these factors to the ability of lower participants to obstruct, there is obviously a more constructive perspective. This unacknowledged power can be (and mostly is) used creatively.

The essential management task may not be to bring the informal distribution of power into line with the formal structure, but rather to acknowledge the inevitability of unofficial influence of the staff farther down the line and create conditions where their power is used for innovation and not to obstruct change. There is one obvious immediate implication for those who manage them. Since we have identified them as potential and actual innovators with considerable authority, the rather charitable notion of 'consultation' may be insufficient to create these conditions. Negotiations may be a more appropriate way.

An acknowledgement of their power by senior management or recognition in formal descriptions of organisational structure may not, however, be sufficient. If health service 'providers' are so crucial to innovation as Donnison and Chapman found that their counterparts in social welfare institutions were, then they must be helped to maximise their contribution. How can this be achieved?

(i) Increasing organisational appreciation. One assumption which underpins this book is that an enhanced understanding of their own organisation will enable managers to be more effective. If this is accepted, then the emphasis in management training should be on helping staff to understand how their organisation actually works. It implies too an introduction to organisational theory early in the career of professional and managerial staff to develop the expertise necessary to maximise their impact on the service.

We have pointed out that people have different abilities and opportunities to innovate. All radiographers, physiotherapists, health visitors and charge nurses have not the same opportunities to promote change. The analysis of the sources of their power will hopefully help them to reach a realistic assessment of what they can hope to achieve. If this is linked with a clearer appreciation of the possible motives of others which will enable them to obtain more co-operation from colleagues, the consequent higher level of co-ordination will represent a real saving in resources which we have postulated as a major goal. Less time spent in achieving co-operation implies a margin of surplus resources available for investment elsewhere.

(ii) Changing the ratio between resources and demand. Innovation does not necessarily mean grandiose projects with regional or national implications. The more practical and limited contributions (e.g. a new way of keeping records which reduces the time spent finding them) are also included. Indeed it is at this level of innovation that many of the extra resources for improvement in services without extra cost will come. And the task of managers (and therefore the responsibility) is to provide these extra resources and improved services to meet higher expectations of staff and public.

Donnison and Chapman's work emphasised the link between innovation and a surplus of resources above formal commitments.[8] This is not only for the seemingly obvious reason that only then can a new service be developed (which may provide compensatory savings elsewhere) but because of the iron law that most of us give routine a higher priority than we do to planning or creative thinking. We know from studies of people in organisations that given a choice between routine day-to-day problems on the one hand, and thinking about a possible problem which may arise in three months, the former will usually be given precedence. If we want the 'creative thinking' to be done by people with day-to-day responsibilities for services, then we must somehow free them from the precedence they normally give to routine.

The change in ratio between resources and demand in favour of the former does not depend necessarily on an increase in resources. Overtime working and increased productivity can also provide the margin. Reducing demand is another alternative.

If this observation drawn from social welfare and other institutions holds good for the health service, then the moral is clear. A proportion of the savings from increased efficiency must be retained by the department if it is one which ought to be encouraged; and these 'savings' should not be absorbed willy nilly by meeting a higher proportion of the demand on that department.

(iii) Persuading those who control the resources. Those who control the resources are involved (or ought to be) in a decision to innovate whether additional resources are required or 'savings' utilised. A problem for the manager is to obtain approval and retain considerable discretion over how the resources will be used. Departmental discretion is conducive to innovation.

Donnison and Chapman describe the process of persuasion thus. 'To gain support of all these people (including controllers) the providers must commit themselves to achieving certain objectives regarded as valuable or acceptable by those controlling the resources . . . The commitments and claims offered as an inducement, to secure resources required at this stage, tend either to be specific but unimportant or important but ill-defined.'[9]

In the development of the centralised emergency chemical pathological service in central London, the support of the controllers (in this case the administrators) might be gained by pointing to the poorer level of analysis under the existing arrangements.[10] They might be further persuaded by facts suggesting that the cost of the centralised service would be lower because of the employment of students. In return the providers could commit themselves to quality checks on the work. This would be an example of a specific but unimportant objective. It would have little impact on their discretionary powers to develop the service in the way they thought best. Or again, they might be asked to ensure rapid processing and reporting to offset the inevitable objections to transporting specimens. If so, this would be an example of an important but ill-defined objective. If commitments of this type are exacted – as they seem likely – the requisite discretion would be left with the staff who provide the service.

All these processes – changing the ratio between provision and resources, persuading the controllers that your investment of the savings is the most productive one, and retaining sufficient discretion over the affairs of the department – require appreciative and manipulative skills of a high order. They require skills not usually developed as part of professional training; nor are they automatically acquired through experience. The right kind of training will help managers to acquire these skills. The assimilation of these skills will indirectly provide the margin of surplus resources which alone can really meet the aspirations of the providers.

III THE RESPONSIBILITIES OF POWER

What would life be like in such an organisation which did these things? Just how much responsibility, for example for innovation, could the health service managers accept? And for what exactly could they be held accountable? We can get some idea of the implications of a system which acknowledged and emphasised their responsibility by reflecting on two cases provided by students on a management course in which the author was involved. The two cases have been edited and simplified for our purposes. They are nevertheless easily recognisable as typical management problems in the health service.

1. *The case of the missing radiographers*
In the course of planning a new hospital the superintendent radiographer designate had been asked for advice on the appropriate establishment for his department. He had suggested a figure of twenty-one. This was in response to an estimate suggesting a workload of 65,000 units. He was later informed the establishment had been fixed at eighteen. About two years after the opening of the department, the actual number of units of work had reached 82,300 per annum.

The superintendent felt that signs of strain within the department were manifesting themselves. In particular, reports were taking longer to produce and the waiting periods for special X-rays were increasing. Naturally this situation concerned both the superintendent and his staff. The superintendent was particularly worried because morale was beginning to sag and as a result retention and recruitment of staff was becoming difficult.

The superintendent, who had felt aggrieved at being asked his opinion on the establishment and then told it was to be three less than his figure, saw as a partial solution to his problem an increase in establishment figures. This would permit a greater number of senior posts to entice staff to the area and perhaps help to retain them. He solicited the support of the radiologist who, however, proved indifferent to his entreaties. The superintendent felt him to be uninterested in organisational matters. An approach to the hospital secretary was received slightly more sympathetically but equally unhelpfully. The superintendent was told any request for an increase in establishment would have to come via the radiologist. His support would be crucial. Further attempts to enlist the support of the radiologist failed.

The superintendent's reaction was inevitable. 'What is the use of trying – they won't listen!' One initial reaction had been to let the service go to pieces, but he quickly rejected this course of action as unprofessional. The patient must not be the one to suffer. He was critical too of the administration 'who must have known' from the statistics supplied to them of the increasing workload. Yet they had not taken any initiative in raising the matter.

This was the point the issue had reached when the superintendent raised the matter for discussion between members of the course. In discussion there were many points raised about the symptoms of strain in the department, man management, communications, and the possibilities of recruitment. Our concern here, however, is more restricted. It centres on one question and its corollary – what could the superintendent do to press his solution? And what kind of action should be expected of him?

There were a number of alternative courses of action open to the superintendent:

(a) Do nothing, say nothing and try to cope with the situation. This was an acceptance of the increasingly unsatisfactory status quo as far as the superintendent was concerned.

(b) Put more pressure either on the radiologist and/or the hospital secretary by additional attempts at persuasion while trying to maintain the service at its present level.

(c) Put more pressure either on the radiologist and/or the hospital secretary, and in the meantime insist on a reduction in the standard of service.

The superintendent had opted for the second course of action. The disadvantage of this option was the continuing strain of offering a service in what he strongly felt was a deteriorating situation. He felt pessimistic about the chance of obtaining a favourable response from the radiologist and hospital secretary, and there was no other person in the organisation who was likely to be able to help. The course gave him the opportunity to raise this in the presence of a senior group officer who was involved in a teaching capacity. Since the issue was raised as a case study for teaching purposes it did not constitute a direct approach which may have posed problems of protocol and jeopardised subsequent relationships within the hospital. In the event, he was again referred to the radiologist! Another disadvantage of this type of continual pressure is illustrated by the negative impact of a nagging wife.

The third option was the more abrasive one, and to be employed only if the departmental head was convinced of the merits both of his case and his solution – an increase in establishment. If this type of pressure is to be effective, the effective block has to be identified (radiologist) and the most effective sanction employed. We were told that the radiologist disliked having to say 'no' to his colleagues. If so, a firm stand by the radiographers that certain things would not be done or be done more slowly may have been sufficient to move the radiologist. A substantive plan for rationing demand on the department may have sufficed to gain the radiologist's support for an approach to senior management. This would be more likely if it was tactfully but firmly made clear to him that the alternative would be upsetting to his colleagues because the level of service generally would deteriorate.

We now move from the particular to the general. Two questions of responsibility require consideration. First, what was the responsibility of a hospital secretary in this kind of situation? If the department's morale was declining because of too great a workload, should the hospital secretary have taken the initiative and discussed this with the radiologist? One thing is clear. It is unrealistic to expect the secretary to take dramatic initiatives on the basis of regular statistics. Unless things are brought forcibly to his attention, he must assume it is not a problem which requires his attention. This view may be denounced as advocacy of 'crisis management'. But given our view of the hospital, with departmental staff being the important element in innovation and senior management being more passive, this seems inevitable. Those who control the resources are rather like a fire engine: they are courts of appeal, and legitimisers of the changes already *de facto* introduced in the day-to-day running of the service. To expect them both to innovate and control is perhaps expecting too much of them.

Second, had the department's service deteriorated, and the third course of action not been taken by the superintendent, what blame should attach to him? In our view the answer is a considerable amount. We have said that the nature of hospital organisation means that the administrator can hardly be accountable for breakdowns in service departments if he has not been forcibly forewarned. Again, too, if the radiologist is not interested in organisational matters, then much of the responsibility for getting something changed must rest with the superintendent radiographer. In a situation of this type, a departmental head who had not submitted proposals for rationing the service before a breakdown occurred[11] could be held to have acted ineffectively, and therefore must bear a large part of the responsibility.

2. *The case of the defective bedpan steriliser*

A thirty-bedded medical ward was blessed with a defective bedpan steriliser.[12] The chief complaint was the frequency with which the front piece fell forward of its own volition. The charge nurse not unnaturally felt this an unnecessary hazard for his students and staff. Frequent repairs by the manufacturers only made for temporary improvements. The inspectors from the General Nursing Council had commented on the need for a new bedpan steriliser after one of their visits. It was agreed that a new one was required.

For two consecutive years a new bedpan steriliser was included in the preliminary estimates, but on both occasions was deleted. The number of patients confined to bed on the ward was small and thus the priority was low. The charge nurse saw his role to be three-fold. First, by warnings and special care he hoped to avoid accidents. Second, to press his claim for a new steriliser. Third, he felt it was his responsibility to explain to staff why they had to put up with a defective steriliser for so long. Since demand for resources outstripped supply, there had to be rationing and there were higher priorities than a new bedpan steriliser for the medical ward.

The affair remained in this sub-acute stage until the staff nurse complained to him that a new carpet and hand-painted wallpaper had been provided in the new office of the hospital secretary. The charge nurse was chided for lecturing them on priorities! He was asked whether he agreed that a carpet and hand-painted wallpaper were a higher priority than a new bedpan steriliser.

Again we look at the issue from the viewpoint of the ward staff who would be perhaps unimpressed by an argument that it was difficult to transfer income between subheads. If for no other reason than the morale of his own staff, the charge nurse had to renew his pressure. The staff felt let down and argued that they had been treated unfairly. But what more could he do? Courses of action open to the charge nurse suggested by other course members included:

(1) Diligent recording of all accidents, including minor ones, caused by the bedpan steriliser. It was felt that unlike routine statistics, a sudden spurt of accident reports (particularly if they were reported to committee) would capture the attention of the hospital administrators, who, for this type of expenditure and decisions on priority, are the controllers of resources.

(2) Ensure that all visitors to the ward, e.g. committee members, inspectors, saw the sluice room and that the defective steriliser was brought to their attention.
(3) Refuse to use the steriliser. This would ensure the attention of the administrators because in the absence of a replacement some sharing arrangements would be necessary. The disadvantages of this course of action (and to a lesser extent (2)) were the effect on the personal standing of the charge nurse in the opinion of the people who would write his reference should he seek promotion. There was also the impact of militancy on future relationships.

In fact, the major problem may not have been the steriliser *per se*, but the feeling of injustice among staff. A combination of options (1) and (2) might have been sufficient to maintain the position of the charge nurse with his subordinates without running the risk of being branded as a 'trouble-maker' by his seniors. The choice between loyalty to one's juniors or seniors is a subject to which we return in a later chapter.

This brief description indicates there were things the charge nurse could do to achieve his objective. His influence was not spent by abortive efforts to get the sterilizer included in the estimates. For what then could we hold the charge nurse responsible? Had there been either an accident or difficulties with ward staff, we could reasonably hold him partially responsible had he not pushed his case further.

In both cases we could hold the departmental heads accountable for any serious breakdowns had they not used their power and influence to the full. The level of responsibility this implies is far greater than normally ascribed in formal descriptions of the role of managers at this level.

This kind of responsibility may not be welcome. There is a strong preference for scapegoats. There are also the obstacles of the tradition, particularly in nursing, which emphasises adherence to rules and discipline and the possibility that some semi-professional groups do not want the responsibilities that accompany full professional status. In these circumstances an acknowledgement of responsibility for innovation, together with higher expectations of their performance in securing co-operation and man management, may not be altogether welcome. Again where there is uncertainty and anxiety more explicit definitions of responsibilities may also be unwelcome.

We turn to the problem of motivating staff later. We may be

encouraged, however, by the fact that Donnison and Chapman are describing what *does* happen. In their studies, social welfare workers did play a large part in innovation. Obviously too some health service providers do so now. The problem is to motivate those who do not now see themselves in this role to use their power to improve efficiency in order to produce the additional resources required for development.

There are obvious implications in this argument for those who control the allocation of resources, too. First, they too have to find ways of motivating other managers to seek and accept responsibility for initiating change among other things. And second, they perhaps have to accept a more restricted view of their own role. *They* are not the sole agents of change. Those controllers who see themselves as the innovative and decisive force of the organisation may find it difficult to accept that leadership in some respects comes from below.

We now have a clearer answer to the question of power and responsibility in the health service. Those who run the service have considerable power in its development and growth. It is they too who have to face up to the problem of more service out of limited resources.

12

Efficiency in the Health Service

If those who provide the service have more power to obstruct and innovate than is usually acknowledged, improvements in the quality of care should flow from a more effective use of their contribution. This depends not only on a recognition of that power and an acceptance of the responsibility that goes with it, but a realisation that the improvements have to be sought within present resources and organisational constraints. We now turn to the contribution those who manage the service can make to increased efficiency.

We separate out the problems of efficiency and man management. This is partly to make the material more manageable. Another reason is that 'good' personnel management is not always synonymous with efficiency in the way we shall use the term. However, better staff management is clearly part and parcel of any drive to increase efficiency.

WHAT IS EFFICIENCY IN THE HEALTH SERVICE?

Often efficient management means little more than 'good management'. We need to be more specific. Elkin and Cornick have defined efficiency as 'The ratio of the quantity of units produced from a system to the quantity of units put into the system'.[1] If we take this definition as our starting point it is clear that they are not talking directly here about the effectiveness of the service. Effectiveness is a measure of the degree to which the service reaches its objectives, while the definition is concerned with the *ratio* of input to output, and how to change it in the direction of greater output from a given level of resources. They are talking about the *means* of improving the service.

Simon's description of the principle of efficiency takes us a little further: '. . . among several alternatives involving the same expenditure the one should always be selected which leads to the greatest accomplishment of administrative objectives; and among

103

several alternatives that lead to the same accomplishment the one should be selected which involves the least expenditure.'[2]

Efficiency has at least two elements; doing more for the same input or less and a rigorous scrutiny of alternative investments. There must be a conscious choice of priorities to establish which development would produce the greatest benefit. Both elements – efficient investment and the efficient day-to-day use of resources – are included in our definition.

There is an immediate objection with which we must deal. Can such a concept of efficiency be given the pre-eminence in health service decision-making as we have suggested it must? Or is such a concept or concepts inappropriate? Judgements about efficiency imply agreement on objectives. Otherwise against what standards can performance be measured? Without such measures can one talk about efficiency sensibly? There are no easy answers to this objection. We have talked already of the difficulty of deciding what are the objectives of the health service. There is the additional problem of devising suitable units for measurement of inputs and outputs. Both difficulties in turn give opportunities for more alibis when questions are asked of current management performance. I well remember accompanying a regional hospital board treasurer on visits to management committees to discuss the annual costing returns. It was quite dispiriting. All except one or two of the variations between the costs of the hospitals which were the subject of the enquiry and those at other hospitals were explained in terms of 'defective' statistics or 'special circumstances'. There were sufficient doubts about the measures being used to provide an alibi for the officers of the management committee if it preferred not to be self-critical and dissatisfied with its own performance.

Yet we are asking that judgements as to whether a service is operating at a satisfactory level of efficiency and the investment which will produce the greatest benefit be made more rigorously. The chairman of the advisory committee on management efficiency, quoted with approval by Spencer, suggested a way out of this dilemma in respect of hospitals:

'. . . it might be that the real question we want to answer is "is this hospital clearly good, or clearly inferior in some respect or another?" – on the principle that wanting to make this judgement is only preliminary to doing something about it, and that on first appraisal only the peaks and hollows are important – the question of whether the general levels of achievement are adequate comes later.'[3]

Simon also sees the problem as a choice in decision-making between the criteria of efficiency and adequacy.[4] In the health service, particularly since those who use the resources are divorced from the process of raising them, there will always be a concern with what is an adequate service. The budgeting game and the professional's desire to provide the best possible service combine to make the criteria of adequacy the major influence in decision-making. What needs to be changed is the balance between the two criteria. More emphasis must be given to considerations of efficiency.

Clearly there are difficulties. Yet a greater willingness to be influenced by considerations of efficiency and look for the 'peaks and hollows' of performance is the way to produce those resources which so many in and out of the service want.

So far this has been a general discussion. We now look at two actual examples of decision-making, which will figure in subsequent discussions, to make our concept of efficiency clearer. They are both drawn from the experience of the author, though they have been amended slightly for this purpose. They have a strong basis in fact.

THE CRITERION OF EFFICIENCY IN DECISION-MAKING

Illustration 1 – The case of the cold food

The problem of cold food for patients is not a new one. In the early 1960s the author met the economic director of a continental hospital who had made a systematic attempt to overcome the problem.

He explained how staff (mostly nuns) and patients had complained that the food was too cold when delivered to the wards or staff canteen. Since the complaints were persistent and had an obvious basis in fact, the director decided that he must remedy this. He started by initiating a thorough analysis. The temperature of the food was taken at various points in the process of preparation and delivery. Since the investigation showed that the major heat loss was not during transit from the kitchen to the ward or canteen, electrically heated trolleys were not the answer. The major heat loss occurred during preparation in the kitchen. The director felt the only effective remedy to this problem was a reorganisation of kitchen equipment and routines which would allow food to be cooked later and processed more quickly. This would involve extensive alterations which would cost a considerable amount of money.

The director rejected the obvious solution of increasing tariffs for this purpose. For one thing it would involve a detailed investigation of the hospital finances by representatives of central government before an increase was approved. In a hospital which prized its independence this scrutiny was not welcome. If this were to be avoided, at least part of the necessary resources would have to come from internal savings. But from what services?

Since the staff had joined in the complaints and therefore seemed to consider warmer food a high priority the economic director was able to put the onus back on to them to find the necessary savings. What were they doing at the moment which could cost less to do or alternatively had a lower priority than warmer food? Each head of department was faced with this question. They had to compare what they were doing against an improvement which they agreed was needed. By this process funds were found to pay for the improvements in the kitchen.

I was taken on a tour of the hospital and asked to taste the food on the wards. I was able to confirm that the reorganisation of the kitchen was a success! The number of complaints about cold food fell dramatically.

THE CRITERION OF EFFICIENCY IN DECISION-MAKING

Illustration 2 – The case of the surplus stenographers
A company offered to install a temporary central dictation system in a small hospital free of charge. This was not only to boost sales; the company was also trying to pre-empt rivals and establish goodwill in a group which was soon to have a new general hospital.

The offer was made at an opportune time. Plans for the new hospital were well advanced which made 'experiments' of this type valuable and the consultants had again recently complained about the inadequacy of the existing medical stenographer service. The medical staff readily agreed to have this central dictation system installed on an experimental basis because it held out the promise of a better service.

The system was quickly installed. It consisted of a telephone handset which was separate from the telephone system, with a central recording mechanism. There were a number of features which attracted the consultants. Recordings were made on to separate discs which could be filed away for future reference. It was also possible for a consultant to call the stenographers' office via the dictation system to indicate to a particular stenographer that he was about to record. In this way it was possible to ensure that the typist most conversant with the terminology of his speciality did the typing.

The service was a popular one. Medical staff in the outpatient department were the heaviest users of the system and only one consultant insisted on dictating directly to a stenographer. The occasions when it was impossible to dictate because the system was fully engaged were rare. The only rumblings of discontent came from the stenographers because of their lack of opportunity to practise shorthand.

After the trial period the company wrote a report on the experiment. The discs were available to calculate the amount of typing actually done during the trial period: allowances were made for work not arising from the central dictation system. On a very conservative estimate the estimate of workload made two typists redundant. This was after a most generous allowance for sickness and holidays and a lower workload than what the company insisted was normal in commercial undertakings. In theory the managers and providers had at their disposal a potential £1,500 (early 1960 salary scales) in savings.

At this time the pathologist, with the support of other medical staff was considering the introduction of a limited diagnostic cytology service. By rearrangement of duties within the pathology department and retraining of existing staff, it was felt this could be satisfactorily provided with the additional appointment of one student laboratory technician. It was thought that funds would be made available for this appointment in the following year's estimates which were still some months away.

It was suggested informally that the resources saved by the central dictation scheme, now installed on a permanent basis, could be used to fund the employment of a student laboratory technician somewhat earlier than planned. This idea for alternative investment was not pursued partly on the grounds that additional money would be forthcoming for the additional student laboratory technician and partly on the grounds that the retention of the two posts in the medical stenographers' department would enable them to offer a 'better service'.

There was no real attempt to evaluate the greater benefit to be gained from the £1,500 ('we don't operate like that') partly because of the difficulties involved in any change. It is much easier to retain the status quo.

THE CASE STUDIES AND THE DEFINITION OF EFFICIENCY

The illustrations are not offered in any anti-chauvinistic way. They happen to be good examples of the attitudes of particular administrators at a particular time to the efficient use of resources. There are examples of both approaches in all countries. It might also be argued that the options open to the economic director were greater than would be open to his counterpart in the United Kingdom. He did not have to struggle with the problem of virement and the distinction between revenue and capital expenditure was far more flexible.

In spite of these reservations the two studies illustrate the important differences in *attitude* towards the efficient use of resources. In the first example the director raided departmental budgets to fund a much-needed improvement. Since some of the pressure for the improvement had come from the staff, they could legitimately be asked to share some of the responsibility for finding the resources to fund it. It was up to them to maintain services within their diminished budgets by increased efficiency. They were asked, too, to decide on the most profitable investment of resources.

In the second example there was less challenge, partly perhaps because the initiative for change had come from senior management. They would have found it more difficult to challenge a head of department to justify the retention of the £1,500 per annum in the departmental budget. The absence of a critical examination to decide the most beneficial investment of the surplus resources is, however, the crucial distinction between the two cases. The second illustration demonstrates the concept of adequacy – what do they need and what should they have – at work in decision-making.

13

Management Techniques and Efficiency

So much for a more precise definition of efficiency. Unfortunately, definitions are not in themselves the spur to action. The problem of motivating those in the service to behave accordingly remains. There are, however, management tools available to help staff assess their performances and hopefully make them seek to improve them. A number immediately spring to mind but we will limit discussion to the following three: (a) management information; (b) management by objectives; (c) correct allocation of decision-making.

I MANAGEMENT INFORMATION AND THE CRITERION OF EFFICIENCY[1]

An important objective for management information is to encourage the provider to be self-critical. This was the reasoning, for example, behind the management audit sponsored by the King's Fund. A checklist of good management practices was circulated to hospital authorities to encourage self-examination.[2]

There is now a wealth of management information available to encourage comparisons of performance. Perhaps the most extensive are the annual hospital costing returns. Reformed in 1966, the scheme now provides regional, national and hospital costs on a uniform basis for all hospitals. Since the departmental costs are largely those arising within the department there can be less criticism of being held responsible for levels of expenditure over which the head or staff of the department have no control.

Many of the doubts about the validity of the units, particularly in the pathology departments, persist, thus undermining the impact of the figures. There are more serious criticisms. Feldstein has argued the measures of output used are none too helpful. The cost per case, for example, is a poor measure of hospital performance. The types of cases within wards nominally in the same speciality can be widely different. To overcome this objection he prefers a costliness index based on the particular case mix, and using the predicted value of what the costs should be.[3] It removes one argument against the official scheme that 'Like is not compared with like'. His is a more refined measure of output and therefore more acceptable for comparisons of performance. If this is a more acceptable basis for comparison of performance then his costliness index can be used to demonstrate the efficiency with which hospitals use the inputs of resources. It is worth reminding ourselves again that in his studies only about one-third of inter-hospital variations in cost per case can be explained by case mix differences. Much of the remaining balance must be due to different levels of efficiency.[4] Work of this calibre clearly demonstrates the potential of costing as an aid to efficiency.

The flaws in the existing scheme are recognised by the government. 'The new costing scheme was thus mainly a "tidying-up" operation with fairly limited objectives and there is still room for further development if costing is to play its full part in hospital management . . .'[5]

We can look forward to more helpful analyses. And if we remember that the information in the present costing returns is an *aid* to efficient management, it adequately serves the purpose of widening horizons beyond one's own pastures. It serves to identify the peaks and hollows for the diligent manager.

This judgement that the *existing* costing returns can be a spur to efficiency is reinforced by Montacute's inquiry into the efficiency of the costing schemes operating before April 1966. 'In general it can be fairly claimed therefore that cost consciousness has increased particularly among "informed" members and staff . . .'[6] He found evidence of savings of a continuing kind, particularly in the catering services.[7]

In altering perceptions of efficiency and indicating where, broadly speaking, a self-examination might be profitable, costing is a valuable aid. Whether it is used as such depends on motivation. 'But it seems there will always remain a "hardcore" . . . Who perhaps due to age, background, prejudice, lack of knowledge or standard of ability are not prepared to be converted . . . it will be these people who continue to hide behind the objections of "too late", "too much paper", "too simple", "too costly", "too blunt".'[8] For those alive to the message of salvation through more efficiency the costing reforms are a useful aid to management.

Another important source of comparative material is the

efficiency studies published by the Department. In this we include the abstract of efficiency studies of the hospital service, hospital abstracts, the hospital activity analysis, and hospital equipment information. A more substantial document is the guide to good practices in hospital administration.[9] The compendium of yardsticks and norms is sufficiently specific for the manager to measure his department's performance over a range of criteria. It provides more specific signposts for him. It also makes interesting reading for those who believe efficiency could be improved. It refers to a review of portering work which reduced standby time from 63·5 to 30 per cent.[10] Or in the department of physical medicine:

'. . . Studies have shown that among other things there is a danger of a high incidence of under-utilised time . . .'[11] 'From a series of studies the conclusion was drawn that significant improvements, possibly of the order of 15 per cent, are generally possible in transport services, mainly by improving journey co-ordination and better control over the use of vehicles and drivers.'[12]

Or in the outpatient department '. . . As little as 7 per cent of qualified nursing staff time has been found to be spent on nursing work . . .',[13] etc. By suggesting yardsticks by which to measure and compare his own performance the diligent member of staff is given excellent tools to assess his own efficiency and indeed indicate how it may be increased. The major contribution is to our first element in efficiency; it indicates where savings may be found. It does not directly help in the second element – the investment of savings to produce the most valued return.

We have talked so far only of the influence of inter-hospital comparisons on perceptions of efficiency. Comparisons of personal performance over time are also important. They are less bedevilled by criticisms of inappropriate bases for comparison. Some of the information collected for the Department on services for patients and the various staff returns can be utilised for this purpose. Had this been done more often it would not have required a special study to discover that the number of stokers had not diminished with the installation of an automatic stoker![14] Another useful source is additional local financial and statistical information made available by the treasurers.

Comparisons of performance between local health authority services before reform were far more problematical. Differences between councils were, or at least were thought to be, even more substantial than those between hospital authorities. The Department of Health and Social Security did give local health authorities 'yardsticks of adequacy in particular services' though the same circular acknowledged they fell 'well short of producing "standards" and "norms" for general application'.[15]

There are three other problems with management information which merit separate mention at this stage. Two stem from the very bulk of the information. First, is there time to read it? Not, of course, if the senior administrator feels he ought to read it first in the belief that initiative for change comes primarily or exclusively from him. The right person to see this type of information is the head of department. He is the one who needs to be convinced that performance should and can be improved. He is in the best position to introduce effective changes.

Second, the provision of management information does not lead to increased efficiency by itself. There is sometimes no realisation that such information is for better management of one's own resources. It is regarded as information for *others* or as advice of 'grandmother telling us how to suck eggs' variety ('What do the *Department* know about health services?'). A report on the response of a sample of hospital authorities to the circular on the management of out-patients was not encouraging. Of the thirty groups only nine had an approach to it which could be called positive.[16] The hospital thought the report revealed 'a comedy of mismanagement'.[17] It is non-action on management information, in this case in the form of circulars, that has necessitated the pink circular routine and, rather unpalatably for hospital staff, an increased emphasis on regional responsibility for managerial performance. Information has to be supplemented in some way with sticks and carrots.

The third objection to measures of performance is the distorting effect on priorities. The provision of quantitative yardsticks and norms of good practice, may lead to too little attention being given to aspects of the work where no such standards exist. One HMC secretary told how as a hospital secretary he had been responsible to the treasurer for some of his work which had been subject to audit. He felt this part of his work had received a disproportionate share of his time and resources.[18]

In spite of these reservations and the absence of uncontroversial measures of output much management information is useful. It can be used to signpost the way to savings and efficient investment. It is valuable if managers are thus made more dissatisfied with present levels of performance and it is seen to be relevant to them rather than the next man. It must also be made available to those in the organisation who can best effect change. The main danger to management information is its champions. It is useful as a guide but not as a basis for hard-and-fast rules.

II MANAGEMENT BY OBJECTIVES AND THE CRITERION OF EFFICIENCY

Decision-making is hampered by the absence of a clear-cut hierarchy of objectives. It is further hampered by what Simon has called the 'bounded rationality' of those who make the decisions.[19] The decision-maker is unable to comprehend all the alternatives or evaluate their probable outcomes so he is unlikely to select the course of action which is the very best in all the circumstances. Accordingly he seeks the solution which 'satisfices' rather than 'maximises'.[20] A system of management by objectives bypasses some of these problems or at least minimises them, and thus opens the way for more decisions informed by the criterion of efficiency.

It bypasses these problems by establishing intermediate goals to guide decisions. These goals, if approved by fellow decision-makers, can be assumed for practical purposes to be consistent with the overall objectives of the service. The objectives provide the much-needed reference point for decision-making. Since the goals are (or can be) devised collectively, there is some pressure for more optimal solutions to problems. They also provide criteria by which performance can be judged, which should act as an incentive to improve performance.

Clearly the type of goals which are chosen are crucial. From our point of view, goals that will enhance efficiency and produce a better return for roughly the same level of input should be given greater priority.

We hasten to add that management by objectives does not solve all the problems of decision-making! They do not, for example, provide yardsticks to judge existing levels of efficiency. They provide rather yardsticks for measuring future performance, though evidence of a low level of previous performance will no doubt influence the choice of objective.

This is a management technique still growing in popularity among managers. In what ways is it applicable in the health service? Or is it applicable? We try to answer these questions by first looking at two examples of management by objectives suggested by people in the service. The first example is taken from a report on an exercise at a management course at the Administrative Staff College where members selected a key area of their own job and defined a target.[21] It is reproduced below:

Key result area	Target (and detailed steps involved)	Control information	Notes
Number of attendances at out-patient department	A REDUCTION IN WAITING TIME IN THE OUT-PATIENT DEPARTMENT FROM THE LAST ASSESSED AVERAGE OF 24 MINUTES TO 12 MINUTES: TO BE ACHIEVED WITHIN THE NEXT NINE MONTHS.		Cost = £1,000 p.a.?
	Among several courses of action, one step will be to appoint a higher clerical officer to carry out regular checks on the operation of the appointment system in the out-patient department, and to survey the problems of waiting there and in the other departments to which out-patients are referred. This person would be on the hospital secretary's staff, and the holder would have a close working relationship with the medical records officer, out-patients sister and the appointment staff.	Job description to be prepared, defining relationship with other staff.	
	1. Consult medical records officer on the present situation and advise him of the proposal to appoint an officer to survey the clinics: request co-operation guidance and assistance. Stress the need for O.P. department staff to work closely with the new officer.		
	2. Discuss the proposal with senior medical staff and clinic staff, presenting the development as a means of	All consultations to be concluded within three weeks of 'go-ahead'.	

obtaining greater efficiency and enabling more patients to be treated.

3. Advise two neighbouring hospitals for whom clinics are held; indicate desire to include their clinics in the surveys.

4. Proceed with appointment, by advertisement if necessary, but preferably from within the organisation.

Response rate; cost.

5. Arrange induction of appointee, and for a period of familiarisation in O.P. procedures and routines of the various clinics (first two weeks).

6. Agree programme of investigation with senior staff concerned and with officer (within one month of starting).

7. Follow-up as necessary throughout year with medical records officer, outpatient sister, senior medical staff and heads of departments.

(a) Fortnightly meetings with officer to receive reports on clinic performances and the need for improved arrangements.

(b) Routine reports to be submitted to medical staff and house committee indicating improvements made and the need for further action.

This particular example was chosen because it is an area of management for which those who provide the services are clearly responsible.

We must bear two maxims in mind while we discuss this and subsequent examples. First, the objectives should be in writing and must be 'statements of precise actions to be taken to achieve the specified results within a given period of time by individual managers'.[22] More general objectives will not achieve the anticipated results (or are less likely to do so). Second, the process of selecting a key area and setting targets for improved perform- ance must be followed by a control mechanism. Senior officers must check targets are being met.

The key to the success of this particular programme is twofold. First, an acceptance by the staff concerned that this is an im- portant objective for which they may have to change their ways if it is to be achieved. Step two is designed to achieve this. Second, the additional information made available by the higher clerical officer will be sufficiently persuasive to achieve changes in pro- cedure. Ways to bring this information to the notice of the decision-makers are specified.

An important element in this example is the assumption of responsibility by the secretary. It is from this decision that the extra cost – an assistant to do the detailed work for him – stems. An alternative strategy of an assumption of responsibility, say by the out-patient sister, who in turn was helped to delegate some routine work, may have been less costly. In many situations it may be a more effective strategy too.

It follows from this assumption of responsibility that the ob- jective of reducing waiting time by 50 per cent in nine months is an incentive for the secretary and the higher clerical officer. Unless it is achieved it will be an adverse reflection on the secretary's managerial ability. And the obstacles – for example the absence of commitment on the part of other staff and the means of persuasion – have to be clearly identified, and thus form sub-objectives for the secretary. He knows what he has to do and how long he has to do it. This is the merit of the technique – the secretary knows the standard against which he will be measured, which provides the incentive; the formulation of the process provides the tactical plan.

What is less clear from this example is the accountability and responsibility of other staff. In what sense will they be held re- sponsible for any failure to meet the target? The alternative strategy would have involved asking the staff actually running the clinic to specify their sub-objectives within the general framework i.e. the reduction of waiting time in nine months.[23] Had this tactic succeeded other staff would have been responsible for the improvement and would have been accountable had the objective not been reached. Their motivation may have been enhanced and their contribution more clearly delineated.

Whatever strategy was adopted, the argument for clearly stated objectives in the health service holds good. An improvement was deemed desirable and the exercise provided the standards against which performance could be judged, delineated responsibility and accountability and thereby hopefully enhanced motivation. And clearly staff are involved both in initiation and successful execution: if done properly it will improve their standard of performance.

The second example is from a clinical setting and is designed to strengthen the point about general applicability and relevance of management by objectives to the health service. The particular example is at far too general a level for it to fall into the province of those who are responsible for day-to-day management though it would involve them setting their own sub-objectives for its achievement. It has been chosen, however, because it demonstrates management by objectives in a clinical setting. The example is a general one used for illustrative purposes by Professor W. W. Holland at the IHA conference in 1971. It is not therefore a formalised or finalised example of management by objectives.

Professor Holland took the problem of chronic bronchitis as his illustration of what management by objectives might involve. The objective (admittedly idealistic and probably unachievable)

'is to keep all chronic bronchitics in some sort of work until their normal retiring age. The target that we intend to achieve within a time scale, that is by 1990, is to introduce a form of treatment for all chronic bronchitics. It implies working out a scheme for treatment. It implies providing adequate work space. It implies providing adequate nurses. It implies providing adequate hospital beds so that we can care for the individual chronic bronchitic when he needs admission into hospital during an acute episode. This implies that we have to allocate the resources available so as to give the best choice between these various possible methods. For example, we may find that it is better to care for the chronic bronchitic within his own home during an exacerbation, rather than admit him to hospital. We may find that it is better to ventilate properly and get rid of pollution in the long-stay wards of hospitals rather than in the acute-stay wards of a hospital where a patient will only be a few days. This will involve building and other programmes and the allocation of adequate drug therapy, and finally again, all the time, it will require research as to the effectiveness of the various forms of therapy and management and the methods of delivery of these.'[24]

For those involved in the care and treatment of chronic bronchitis such an exercise would provide some of the objectives to guide decision-making. The purpose of the treatment would be clearer and a basis for judgement of performance would be provided. And we can assume, as in the previous example, that the setting of targets would provide an incentive to improve performance.

There are three obvious implications. First, if the technique is to be applied to clinical objectives choices have to be made between alternative courses of action rather than backing both horses: this would be a painful exercise and involve disruption of existing patterns of care. Second, those in the service would be involved; sub-objectives for participants would have to be specified and a time scale agreed. Third, the estimate of costs to achieve this objective would be a claim on future resources and on savings produced by greater efficiency.

Both examples show the applicability of the technique in the health service. Both, however, would have increased effectiveness rather than increased output or gained greater value from existing resources, and it is the latter process which will produce the extra resources for improvements in service. We now need to consider carefully in what ways the technique could be used to meet our objective of greater efficiency in the more restricted way we have defined it.

We do this by taking a hypothetical example from an area of day-to-day management. We stay in the realms of out-patient departments and clinics. In a large department or clinic a saving of 10 per cent in the time of trained nurses would dispense with the necessity of at least one nurse, and probably more. The nurse would then be available for service elsewhere. This would be a worthwhile objective, and one that could be promoted by the nurse manager in charge. Let us now state a possible objective for the nurse a little more clearly.

Objective: In one year the number of hours worked by trained nurses in the out-patient department or clinic will drop by 10 per cent without reducing the standards of service to the doctor or patient. Any substitution of labour would have to involve a financial saving.

We know this is a realisable objective for many out-patient

departments at least since so little of the trained nurse's time is spent in performing duties requiring her skills. As little as 7 per cent of the trained nurse's time can be spent on nursing duties.[25]

What would such a commitment involve? One of the first steps for the sister or superintendent would be to discuss with her staff how they could so re-schedule their duties to maximise the technical skills of the trained nurse; this in turn would require an examination of the content of work at particular clinics and the times when the skills were required. It might (indeed should) produce a discussion on the movement of patients and how this might be changed to the advantage of staff and patients. A similar analysis would be required for the location of equipment. This process would provide the sub-objectives or targets for staff, a list of the detailed steps involved and the control information required.

This is the basis for a strategy to re-schedule work and reduce the trained nursing work force by 10 per cent. Say, for argument, this became in practical terms the replacement of three full-time nursing staff by two part-time staff and a receptionist within twelve months. The achievement of the objective could entail either (1) waiting for the resignation of full-time staff and replacing them with part-time staff, and/or (2) inquiring whether some staff would like a transfer, and/or (3) inquiring whether some full-time staff might not prefer a part-time job, and (4) arranging the employment of a receptionist and suitable training.

Another very important step would be consultation with the medical staff. Early consultation, simultaneously with that of the nursing staff, might produce openings (e.g. 'Can only trained nurses record the weights of patients?') which might be useful when redeployment of trained staff was discussed. Certainly there would have to be consultations over strategy since medical staff approval or disapproval would be crucial. The medium of consultation – informal or more formal ones with the medical divisions, etc., would depend on the local situation and the superintendent. To use a phrase employed earlier, the 'support and encouragement' of senior staff would be required. It might be useful, or essential, if some structural alterations or additional equipment became part of the strategy.

As a hypothetical example there will be a number of objections. The most important may be the adverse reaction of the medical staff. 'They will insist on trained nurses.' 'We have got to be around all the time to be available just when the doctor needs our help.' This type of constraint which produces insoluble problems may be thought to be one which makes management by objectives less relevant in the health service. However, medical staff may not be as 'monolithic' as they are portrayed to be. There is usually the radical as well as the arch-conservative among them. The challenge of management by objectives is that a strategy has to be adopted which will take such factors into account.

Another objection associated with the first will be the question of accountability. How can the nurse manager be held accountable when so much depends on the co-operation of medical, senior nursing and administrative staff over which she has no hierarchical authority? The achievement of many things depends on the co-operation of others. However, management responsibility does involve ensuring good co-operation. One advantage of management by objectives is the additional pressures it produces to find new ways of achieving the co-operation of others. In this case it may be achieved by convincing doctors that they would receive a better service or even the additional availability of a nurse for a long-cherished project! The administrators, on the other hand, could be encouraged by the prospect of savings. Since these are skills (largely intuitive) which most managers have, arguments that they cannot be expected to be responsible for gaining the co-operation of others should not be given too much weight. In some cases they are obviously valid. What we must do is not to assume them to be so.

Such a project, if successful, could meet our criteria of efficiency in both senses. The reduction of costs for similar input (service) would make additional resources available for investment elsewhere. The criteria for determination of that investment hopefully would be that of efficiency.

All three examples demonstrate the applicability of this technique to health service management, and its usefulness in the drive to increase efficiency. Yet it is not a painless exercise. For example, before any increase in establishment is requested, responsible managers should be expected to exhaust all means of increasing productivity by reorganisation. It follows that managers should be asked for evidence that they had done so before approval for an increase could be given. This may produce a sense of insecurity particularly if it becomes clear that managers no longer have a prescriptive right to existing or previous levels of resources. It would increase the emphasis on planning at the expense of the priority given to the routine demands on time. It would be a very challenging environment.

The technique is more than a formulation of what many staff already try to do informally. It is easy to allow enthusiasm for a new technique to cloud judgement about its real value and expose it to criticisms of gimmickry and 'teaching grandmother to suck eggs'. It is the *formalisation* of the process which is important. This formalisation implies more specific commitments and therefore accountability than hitherto, the identification of possible obstacles and the development of strategies to overcome them. The time limit provides an incentive for action now. There is a contribution to be made by management by objectives to increased efficiency, though much of the merit may be in doing the exercise rather than the exercise itself!

In conclusion we must add that management by objectives is a means of improving performance generally and not, of course, confined to improving efficiency in the narrow way we have defined it. The case for its use is much more widely based than this. Pantall and Elliot, for example, in reviewing their work at the East Birmingham Hospital pointed out that it can lead to 'more real delegation, the removal of fuzzy lines of demarcation, the better choice of revenue priorities, the better choice and development of staff'.[26]

III CORRECT ALLOCATION OF DECISION-MAKING AND THE CRITERION OF EFFICIENCY

A judicious allocation of responsibility for particular decisions enhances the importance of the criterion of efficiency in decision-making. '. . . each decision should be located at the point where it will be of necessity approached as a question of efficiency rather than a question of adequacy. . . . The only person who can approach competently the task of weighing their relative importance is one who is responsible for both or neither.'[27] For those who stand to lose or benefit by the choice it is important, too, that justice must be seen to be done.

In simple terms a decision on what to do with a saving of £1,500 cannot be taken by the head of the department involved. For example, a records officer in a similar position to that described in the case of the central dictation system, no doubt if challenged to say why the money should stay in the department, would think of many justifications for doing so. His reasons would have their main source in notions of adequacy – what does his department need? This is even more likely if the alternative decision meant a switch of funds to another department and posed questions about the value of existing services compared with projected ones. The more important the stakes the greater the difficulties: departmental loyalties become even more important factors. A senior administrator hopefully (but not in the particular case), by being equally interested or disinterested, would be more likely to view the issue from the point of view of efficiency. The records case study reminds us (if it was necessary to do so) that this does not follow automatically.

In the pre-reform service Simon's dictum was probably observed in letter rather than spirit. Those who provided the service had to justify themselves to disinterested or equally interested administrators, treasurers or medical officers of health. Where in the pre-reform hospital service the treasurer and group secretary's departments were involved – for example extra administrative staff – they quite properly had to justify themselves elsewhere. The courts of appeal – under the old hospital system the Regional Hospital Board and the Management Committee – were thus put in a position when the choice could be made on grounds of efficiency. In terms of the Board, for example, would an additional general administrative grade at group X produce more benefit than one at Y group? The health and finance committees were the parallel locus of power in the community health services.

Where the choices lie within the departmental responsibilities the professional manager is the appropriate person to make the decision. His equal interest may lead him to discriminate between the options on grounds of efficiency since notions of adequacy are irrelevant. It should be made clear to him that he is in the best position to choose between existing commitments and desired improvements, too. For example, if the engineer feels a piece of equipment would be of considerable value, he could be told to finance it from savings elsewhere in his department. A decade ago I visited a hospital where the economic manager had been approached by the pathologist for funds to buy an auto-analyser. The pathologist was asked to state his case and in the course of doing so he argued that he could save the time of two technicians if an auto-analyser was purchased. In two years the cost of the auto-analyser would have been covered by savings in staff time. He was taken at his word. The auto-analyser was purchased and the first two technicians to depart were not replaced. There was no additional recruitment until the costs of the auto-analyser had been offset.

How can this distribution of decision-making be developed to ensure that considerations of efficiency are paramount when savings are being allocated or services being evaluated against alternatives? How, for example, could we ensure that managers faced with an alternative investment of £1,500 at present allocated to one department saw it as illegitimate and inefficient to leave it where it was without a thorough evaluation of the benefits accruing from alternative courses of action? Clearly it is not merely a matter of the location of the decision-making, though it is important. Since some administrators already do this, we have to find ways to encourage others to do it as well.

More involvement may help. Collective decision-making makes a number of staff party to a *joint* analysis of the value attached to alternative investments. Needless to say 'value' is a very vague concept: it can, however, be given life by the valuation of particular improvements by joint discussion, agreement or consensus. This is the system which was in effect in many hospital groups for the allocation of improvement monies for medical equipment. The group medical advisory or medical executive committees were often given a specified allocation and the medical staff as equal claimants had to decide the most appropriate distribution. In this way, equally interested parties had to find criteria to discriminate between priorities. And the criterion of efficiency is more likely to be called on to assist in making the allocations.

Collective decision-making in which vested interests have to justify themselves to each other becomes more important the more difficult the decision.

We have talked about the importance of getting decisions about the allocation of the increment and savings in the right place in the organisation. There is a third type of allocative decision. This is weighting the value of existing services against projected improvements. It is this latter type of decision which is clearly the most challenging. Analyses of existing services to establish if there are any which have a lower value than projected improvements is a very threatening process indeed. But there are some who feel such analyses are overdue.

Some, for example, argue that the time, effort and money invested in mass miniature radiography could be more profitably invested elsewhere. Are there not similar examples at a lower level? Tonsils and adenoids? Audits to check correctness of expenditure? Physiotherapy of a 'keep fit' rather than remedial type? Or school health services?

This is the level of efficiency at which senior departmental officials would have liked hospital staff before reform to operate.

'How did the H.M.C.S. deal with their allocations? Did they really examine their priorities each year? Did they concentrate too much on the two and three quarter per cent instead of the whole one hundred and two and three quarters? They should constantly be examining present commitments to see if they could be abandoned or their cost reduced.'[8]

The obvious (and often missed) opportunity for such analyses and greater emphasis on efficiency for all three types of decision is the budgetary cycle. So often in the pre-reform service they were a mathematical exercise with ritualistic overtones which give the impression of a game. 'Ask for twice as much as you want because it will be reduced by 50 per cent anyway. Realistic budgeting – 'we are only going to get two or three per cent more than last year, let's decide what is the most profitable way to spend it,' – may lead to a more critical view of present commitments and more suggestions for improvements. The change in the method of financing of the hospital service in the early years of the decade and budgetary changes in local authorities together with 'forward looks' are excellent opportunities for a change in approach. The latter in particular lift the eyes from the immediate situation and routine problem: they force realisation of the impossibility of financing all improvements from the increment. The promised basis for budgetary allocations to the new health authorities may also serve to undermine the concept of divine right to previous levels of resources. But as with the estimate and budgeting process it depends on the new opportunities being used intelligently. And an intelligent use involves making those who provide the service face the problems of finance, efficiency and evaluating the value of their present services against potential improvements.

It will be important to seize the opportunity presented by integration. The marriage of hospital and community services gives the opportunity to local administrators to compare the value of alternative investments over a wider field. This depends much on the intelligent use of the planning cycle and the operations of the district management teams. The 'representative' nature of some members of the team may encourage comparisons of the value of each other's services. On the other hand, they may not be so equally disinterested as the old management and local health committees were.

This is not a plea for collective decision-making *par excellence*. It is a plea for a shift in decisions about the allocation of resources from the equally disinterested manager (administrator, treasurer) to those who are equally interested. The management teams in the new services provide an excellent opportunity for such a shift.

14

Efficiency in Practice

We have discussed the contribution to efficiency of only three management techniques. There are others which have equally legitimate claims for inclusion. One which is particularly favoured now and to which we have made passing reference is participative management. In our assessment of the prospects for more efficient management of the health service we recognise the contribution of this technique and other unmentioned ones as well as management information systems, management by objectives and reallocation of responsibility on decisions on the use of resources.

It is clear that we cannot expect a transformation in management when these techniques are adopted. For example, we have said collective decision-making on the allocation of resources may give greater weight to considerations of efficiency than a system of detached administrators making the final judgement. However, Pantall and Elliot in their work at East Birmingham found that meetings of heads of departments presented problems. It was not a problem of reticence but the absence of a common interest, 'A meeting . . . though vocal, tends to become the vehicle for the expression of individual departmental grievances rather than for the forging of a common policy.'[1] If this experience were common, or practised where participation was not so genuinely welcomed, would department heads argue in terms of efficiency? On balance probably not. They would argue more probably in terms of 'adequacy' ('We've been short of resources for years – look at our lavatories!'), as the coin of exchange acceptable to them. They would be reluctant, too, to bid for the 'savings' produced in another department (if they were not to be made available to another part of the service). Such a situation would be personally very threatening, since they might feel that they too would soon be in the firing line themselves. As far as the increment was concerned the law of 'buggins turn' might be reinforced. However, a little bit of sun for everybody may not be the most efficient way to invest resources.

Where then does this observation leave the argument for more participation and responsibility in decision-making? Is there any value involving the departmental heads in decision-making? The answer to these questions is that it is worth trying. A start could be made in the allocation of improvement monies (where it hasn't already started). A disinterested party (a senior administrator) could lead the interested parties (heads of departments) to face up to the question of choice *between* services and the criteria on which the choice should be based, and to a more commonly accepted (rather than an official) view of what services or developments should have the highest priority. It might, however, pave the way in time for a more challenging approach to existing commitments and present levels of efficiency.

The increased use of the criterion of efficiency to decide the disposal of savings or to assess the relative value of an existing service compared with a projected development is much more unlikely. Where staff interests are affected adversely it is idealistic to expect them to behave in a purely altruistic way and approach the decision from the standpoint of efficiency.

An illustration will make this point more clearly. A matron of a mentally subnormal hospital, which was fairly well staffed for that type of institution found that she was underspending on nursing salaries. The hospital secretary brought this to her attention. Together they decided she should quickly engage three more staff for the remaining months of the year to ensure the allocation for nursing salaries was taken up. This is a familiar enough situation and a good illustration of the concept of adequacy and departmentalism at work. The former was clearly at work in the feeling that there were never sufficient nurses and that a few more would make the nursing service more adequate. From his account of this event the secretary obviously felt the unspent monies to belong to the nurses and no thought was given to alternative investments. More thought was given to the possibility of losing the equivalent sum in the next financial year or the treasurer regarding this as an underspending which would enable him to keep within the total budget for the group.

More concern for efficiency would have demanded a minimum level action on two counts. First, the matron would have had to justify why the money should be retained for nursing salaries against other desired improvements in the hospital or group. Second, if an alternative investment was considered of greater value (e.g. at another hospital, or employment of other grades of staff) then action should have been taken to get permission to transfer funds. The second outcome could never arise because the first efficiency question – 'Why should *you* have the money, matron?' – was never asked. Getting the matron and hospital secretary to accept the legitimacy of this kind of analysis is going to be a long uphill struggle. It might be fractionally easier if they were expected to justify themselves to other departmental heads who were pressing for additional funds.

However, by making the choices more explicit and presenting them realistically to heads of departments, senior managers may enable them to widen their horizons beyond their particular cabbage patch. A greater loyalty to the wider organisation may in time lead those in the service to search for savings and services of lower value to finance improvements elsewhere – just a *little* more enthusiastically! Given the British way of doing things, this is probably as much as we could hope for from joint discussions among staff on the allocation of resources. Any advance in this direction is, however, worth having.

A cautious judgement of the impact of the other management techniques is also called for. While management information, correct allocation of decision-making on the allocation of resources and management by objectives can help to increase output by improving performance, we must not expect too much. This is particularly so where our two prior conditions do not exist. First, a general acceptance that it is *in*efficient to expect to finance improvements mainly from the increment. Second, staff in the service see they have a contribution to make and use their influence to the maximum effect. When these dicta become part of conventional wisdom more can be expected from management techniques to increase efficiency.

These are the arrows available to the health service manager. At what targets should he aim the arrows?

Moores has rather amusingly listed some examples of inefficiency in the hospital sector. One will suffice for our purpose.

'A large hospital experienced great difficulty in maintaining an establishment of the theatre porters and it was felt that the situation would be eased if a means could be found for producing better work rotas. An examination of what the porters did led to a suggestion that one porter rather than two should control a trolley, and instead of their being assigned permanently to a specific theatre with a consequent utilisation of around 20 per cent they should operate from a pool. The problem then became what to do about nine or ten redundant porters rather than the one originally perceived of how to keep sixteen. At the last reckoning the hospital had managed to secure an increase in establishment to eighteen.'

He ends his recital of this and other examples 'simply due to limitations of space' and points to the 'rationalisations' used to bolster rejection of proposed changes. 'As a taxpayer I am weary of this rationalising . . .'[2] Utilisation of manpower in a labour intensive industry is the obvious place to start in any search for greater efficiency.

PROFESSIONAL STAFF

We have already quoted the conclusion drawn from studies on the use (or misuse) of trained state-registered nurses in out-patient departments. A nursing officer asking for an increase in establishment could reasonably be told that it would be considered when the time spent on skilled nursing duties by trained nurses in the out-patient department had increased by X per cent. Similar comments can be made about other medical auxiliaries. In the departments of physical medicine 'studies have shown that among other things there is a danger of a high incidence of under-utilised time. . . .[3] Personal experience would support this too in radiography departments. The proportion of time spent travelling between patients by those in the community services is another obvious target area for those wishing to increase the use of skilled personnel.

It is not only amongst the medical auxiliaries that greater efficiency should be sought. Medical productivity can be improved. We have already referred to a study whereby reorganisation produced more off-duty time for junior medical staff. Much more ambitious reorganisation, as illustrated in the case of the Kaiser Medical Groups in California, produces even more dramatic increases in available time for investment elsewhere.

'Patients take their own histories with a self-administered questionary and even perform some investigations themselves before seeing the doctor. Results are processed by computer and the physician is presented with a provisional differential diagnosis at his first contact with the patient . . . In this way a great deal of time-consuming and rather tedious medical labour is circumvented. This need not dehumanise medicine . . . for it leaves more time to establish rapport with the patient instead of asking routine questions.'[4]

Some have obviously found increases in medical productivity

possible. Similar concentration on the problem of the 'time expired' registrars at national and regional level would repay the effort.

Efficiency is not, however, necessarily merely doing more of the same thing with the same level of resources. It might involve doing different things. In the example of the Kaiser Medical Groups, allocation of work from doctors to patients and computer left medical staff with 'surplus resources' which they could invest to establish better rapport with patients. On a smaller scale 'the early maternity discharge scheme initiated by Theobald in Bradford actually provided the margin to improve ante-natal treatment and reduce toxaemia deaths'.[5] The value of longer hospital care for maternity patients was judged to be less than improved ante-natal care and a more intensive attack on deaths from toxaemia.

The utilisation of professional manpower can be improved. Not to improve it is inefficient. To improve it is one way to produce the surplus resources required for development.

NON-PROFESSIONAL STAFF

Clearly the same argument applies to the use of non-professional staff. Moores' illustration of inefficient use of porters could be repeated many times as could the abstract of efficiency study on portering work in a Teaching Hospital which reduced the stand-by time from 63·5 to 30 per cent. The same is true of the engineering and building maintenance services.

'Studies have suggested that some maintenance tradesmen are less than 50 per cent effective . . .'[6] Or the provision of hospital transport. 'From a series of studies the conclusion was drawn that significant improvements, possibly of the order of 15 per cent, are generally possible in transport services, mainly by improving journey co-ordination and better control over the use of vehicles and drivers.'[7] These are but three hospital departments. Potential improvements in efficiency are equally available in the others.

The 'guide to good practices' in hospitals is important in that it stresses organisation of work to improve efficiency and not necessarily getting men to work more quickly. The level of efficiency is thus a reflection on the manager's ability to organise.

Interesting too is a comment on how to improve the efficiency of the building and engineering maintenance section. 'A proportion of the work allocated to them is of doubtful value when there are other things of established value to be done.'[8] To be asking for more staff while performing tasks of doubtful value is the epitome of inefficiency.

There are suitable management techniques by which efficiency could be increased in the health service. There are many areas which would repay the application of those techniques. There may be unexpected long-term advantages in doing so. Evidence of greater efficiency may produce a bonus in terms of those extra funds to which providers think themselves entitled. Sir Bruce Fraser, one time permanent secretary to the Ministry of Health is reported as believing 'financial stringency, if it leads to greater efficiency can be the best lever for more money . . . The knowledge that the NHS *is* more efficient will . . . filter upwards and the decision-makers will give the NHS more money because they know the extra funds will be spent wisely.'[9]

More efficient management may not always have a direct financial pay-off in the form of savings. For example, better management in out-patient departments, general practitioner surgeries and clinics will reduce the time lag between appointment and consultation time without necessarily freeing resources for use elsewhere. This incidentally is also a good example of how services can be improved without the input of extra resources.

We have already mentioned some of the obstacles in the path of those pressing for a more efficient use of resources. Perhaps the most important obstacle in the long run is the realisation of how uncomfortable it would be to work in a super-efficient organisation.

At a very practical level heads of departments seeing savings allocated to other departments may be witnessing the departure of staff on whose numbers their own status and salary is based. This fact, of course, militates against the transferring of funds from one department to another on too large a scale, if at all. Since status and power *are* important to staff in the health service a changing environment of this nature might be a nightmare. This would be even more so if an 'organic' system of management developed, leaving considerable obscurities in responsibilities. Too quick a move to organic systems of management (where appropriate) and greater emphasis on efficiency would produce such resistance from staff as to offset most of any advantages so far gained. A balance then has to be struck between the needs of efficiency and reassurance to staff.

In the final analysis, we must remember that it is from present resources that much of the surplus for development to meet rising expectations must be found. If more collective decision-making in the use and allocation of resources moves us only a little way along this path then it is worth while.

15

Value for Staff

More efficient use of resources clearly implies more efficient use of man and womanpower. Since health services are labour intensive, it is the key to improving the level of service within the present constraints on finance and staff recruitment. This is a truism. The difficulties come when discussion turns to the means by which personal productivity can be increased even faster than it has been doing in the past twenty-five years. What help do the various philosophies and techniques of personnel management offer? We explore their value to managers in the health service in this and the next three chapters.

The importance of good staff management as a crucial part of the manager's task cannot be over-emphasised. Indeed, the Brunel researchers have taken responsibility for subordinates as their starting point in the definition of those who can be considered a manager. 'I am going to define manager in a particular way; namely, someone who not only gets work done through others but most importantly, who is *held accountable* by higher authority not only for his own work but also the quality of the work of those others.'[1] (*Author's emphasis*.) This concept of a manager not only underlines the importance of the techniques and philosophies we are about to examine, but it also provides an incentive to better management in that staff are to be held accountable for the quality of the work of their subordinates.

This definition also serves to underline the distinction between our field of interest here and in the previous chapters on efficiency. Here we are concerned with relationships and their management and above all with motivation, while in the previous chapter we concentrated on more impersonal organisational matters. The connecting theme in both is of course better value for resources committed to the health service. One difficulty has to be mentioned at the outset. The definition of efficiency in much of the personnel management literature is less specific than the one we have used. In places 'efficient' is synonymous with 'good' staff management;

and 'good' staff management for some seems to be merely the adoption of current techniques and theories.

The connection between 'good' staff management and efficiency in the way we have previously defined it is not always obvious. This is either because it is difficult to establish the casual connection, say, between good personnel management and higher levels of personal performance or perhaps because there may be none. The different ways of handling and treating employees compared with, say, fifty years ago, owe as much to changing relationships in modern society as to the drive for efficiency. Certainly a manager who wants to maximise efficiency cannot fly in face of what is commonly accepted to be the right way to treat employees. But this is a different argument to the one commonly heard that various man management techniques are *the* way to improve personal performance at work. For these reasons – difficulty of proof, neutral effects and the current beliefs about the 'right' treatment of employees – 'efficiency' in the context of man management often has a less specific meaning than the one we employed in the previous chapter. As a result, we too shall have to talk of 'good' personnel policies. When we do so, however, the reader must bear in mind the narrow definition of efficiency which we see as a major objective for the integrated health service. If at all possible, personnel policies should be judged by this criterion.

In looking at the choices open to the manager, we focus on the problem of motivation. It should be clear, too, from the previous chapter, that the problem is not confined to finding ways to motivate manual workers to achieve a higher level of personal performance, and accept changes in working practices. Non-manual workers will have to improve their productivity too.

We begin by looking briefly at what the employee wants from his employment and what inducements organisations can offer. This provides the groundwork for the discussion in the subsequent three chapters of the various personnel management techniques including, *inter alia*, the place of participative management techniques in the health service.

I   THE EMPLOYEE:
WHAT DOES HE WANT FROM EMPLOYMENT?

This seemingly simple question does not permit equally simple answers. Indeed, one has a wide choice of answers. At one end of the spectrum we have the money theory ('after all, that's what they come to work for, don't they?') – a disarmingly straightforward, no-nonsense explanation. At the other end of the spectrum one has the more complex explanations, offered by theorists like Maslow. He has suggested that people generally are motivated by factors according to a hierarchical arrangement.

the
need
for self
fulfilment
the need for self
expression
the need to belong
the need for physical security, warmth,
shelter, etc.
basic physiological needs such as hunger, thirst etc.[2]

The explanation which the manager chooses often tells us as much about him as it does about the worker. For example, managers who emphasise the importance of financial incentives often couple this with a belief that people do not want to work and are basically lazy. High monetary rewards, discipline and controls are therefore felt to be necessary for maximum output. Managers who, before the return of high unemployment in the late 1960s, referred to the days of unemployment with nostalgia as a means of discipline are an example of this school of thought. No doubt such managers are trying to reconcile their beliefs with the non-impact of high rates of unemployment on the response of employees in the 1970s.

Douglas McGregor of the human relations school naturally sees the problems of personnel management rather differently. 'For management the answer lies in creating such conditions that efforts directed towards the objectives of the enterprise yield genuine satisfaction of important human needs.'[3] A close association between the employee's needs and the job he is asked to do improves recruitment and reduces turnover; and needs are more than just financial ones. Since an employee is only motivated to fulfil a need up to the point of saturation, non-basic ones are likely to become more important in determining the response of the worker.

We have exaggerated the differences between conceptions of

what employees want from work. Most managers fall between these two polar positions with the majority, perhaps, nearer the second. But whatever the manager's view of what the employee wants, it is clear that the interests of the organisation as a whole will preclude these needs being fully satisfied. There is, and must be, give-and-take in the relationship between employees and employers, or the managed and managers.

'The members of an organisation . . . contribute to the organisation in return for inducements that the organisation offers them. The contributions of one group are the source of the inducements that the organisation offers others. If the sum of the contributions is sufficient, in quantity and kind, to supply the necessary quantity and kinds of inducements, the organisation survives and grows: otherwise it shrinks and ultimately disappears unless an equilibrium is reached.'[4]

The objective then is rather to recognise the employee's needs and aim to meet sufficient, not all, of them to retain and motivate him: and to minimise the impact of unmet need and thus potential dissatisfaction on performance.

II   WHAT CAN AN ORGANISATION OFFER?

Let us begin at the level of broad strategies. Galbraith suggests that there are four general means available to organisations to motivate members. One is compulsion – 'failure to accept the goals of the group brings the negative reward of punishment'.[5] Dismissal or even threat of it in a time of great unemployment would fall under this head. So does removal of one's name from the professional register, though in this case the punishment may be initiated by fellow professionals rather than management. In the health services a strategy of compulsion on any scale is unlikely.

Financial incentives are another weapon in the armoury of organisations. In return for money the individual 'offers the organisation . . . undifferentiated time and effort'.[6] In the 1960s the health service saw an increased reliance on financial incentives to achieve some of its objectives. Incentive bonus schemes for manual employees in hospitals and local authorities, overtime and other payments for nursing staff, the 'psychiatric lead' and the inducements to medical staff to work in less popular areas are obvious examples of the use of this form of inducement. Also the presumed association between the staffing difficulties in the health service and low pay is another illustration of how important financial incentives are thought to be by many.

The third type of inducement is identification with the organisation. Simon defines identification with organisational objectives this way: '. . . a person identifies himself with a group when, in making a decision, he evaluates the several alternatives of choice in terms of their consequences for the specific group'.[7] This is the end result of identification with the objectives of the organisation. There are means at the disposal of those who manage to encourage this sense of identification. They may be helped, as Galbraith points out, by the individual concluding that the goals of the group are superior to his own. The promotion of the acceptability of the organisation's goals (and therefore identification) is perhaps a more feasible objective. Development of feelings of identification with the organisation which in turn produces decisions influenced by common goals is perhaps the most important strategy available to the managers in the health service.

Galbraith identifies a fourth type of inducement. He calls this adaptation: '. . . the individual may serve the organisation not because he considers its goal superior to his own but because he hopes to make them accord more closely with his own'.[8] He quotes as an example the 'executive who strings along with much that he thinks routine and unenterprising in the hope of winning support for a new idea of his own'.[9]

Clearly more than one strategy can be pursued at any one time though not all are compatible. The first two inducements 'exist in varying degrees of association with each other',[10] as do identification and adaptation, but these latter strategies can only be combined effectively with financial incentives when the element of compulsion is small. Policies with a large element of compulsion preclude a strategy of increasing motivation through development of a strong sense of identification with an organisation. Conversely, strong commitments to the strategies of identification and adaptation (e.g. by giving more discretion in selected areas) preclude hard-line management.

This very broad description of managerial strategies serves two purposes. First, it helps us to identify those which can be most profitably pursued here. Policy in the health service seems to combine elements of the second and third strategies – financial incentives and development of identification with the organisation. It is on these two strategies that we subsequently concentrate.

Second, they serve to remind managers of the ultimate objectives of such personnel management techniques as job enlargement, staff welfare schemes, participative management, etc. The techniques are not ends in themselves. Their utility should be judged, at least in part, by their contribution to the broad strategies of personnel management.

16

Financial Incentives and Motivation

For managers in the service incentive bonus schemes are perhaps the most obvious way of pursuing this strategy. They are seen as particularly relevant to manual workers. Their introduction is no doubt partly related to the evidence of the wasteful use of their time.

At the time of writing there is no hard evidence of how successful these incentive bonus schemes have been. We have thus to draw on our knowledge of their efficiency in other organisations to reach a considered judgement. The relationship between higher rewards and a higher level of output is not as obvious as some might have us believe. For example, there are some workers who prefer the 'leisure option' to higher earnings. This has been so clearly demonstrated by some miners who, after reaching a financial threshold, prefer to work only four days per week in spite of financial incentives to work five. Again, there is considerable evidence that workers impose restrictions on the level of ouput below the expectations of management even where this produces a financial disadvantage. If workers restrict output to maximise influence then an introduction of an incentive bonus scheme may undermine feelings of security bound up with the familiar, and thus increase the problems of managers who want to increase it. Clearly we must not over-estimate the likely effect of incentive bonus schemes or indeed other features of a financial incentive strategy. This is particularly so in the health service where non-financial motives are probably even more important in determining the response of workers.

These other needs or motives are often underestimated by managers. Rosemary Stewart quotes an industrial study in which workers, foreman and general foreman were asked what satisfactions each most wanted from his job. The two senior grades, the foreman and general foreman were also questioned on what they thought their subordinates wanted. It is these latter expectations which are revealing. 'The supervisors consistently overrated the importance of economic factors to their subordinates and underestimated the importance of social satisfactions, such as getting along well with the people they "work with" and a "good chance to do interesting work." The superiors would have been far more accurate in their estimates of what their subordinates wanted if they had assumed they wanted much the same as they did.'[1] Significantly, one hospital administrator in a brief sketch of reactions to interim bonus schemes has commented: 'Perhaps the purely financial factors in staff motivation have been over-estimated.'[2]

This is more commonly accepted when non-manual staff are involved, though even here inducements have been introduced to attract and retain staff in less popular specialities. Though relevant, they are not seen to be the major contribution in encouraging the non-manual worker to move to a poorer area, accept changes in organisation or work harder. The major contribution comes from identification with the service or a particular employer.

It would be absurd to suggest financial incentives are totally ineffective. It is rather that above a certain level of income they become less decisive in motivation and attempts to enhance motivation with financial inducements may produce as many problems as they solve. It would seem that the key to enhanced motivation and, therefore, higher productivity among employees may lay elsewhere.

'Our brief survey of the search for panaceas to solve all problems of management – labour co-operation shows that there are none. The belief, for instance, that payment by results is the answer to enlisting workers' co-operation in higher productivity is based on too simple a view of human motivation ... The challenge is to provide the conditions in which people will want to work and therefore to co-operate.[3]

This was written many years before the hospital service and local authorities got around to introducing their own incentive bonus schemes.

Another disadvantage of incentive bonus schemes is the unrealistic expectations of them. If they make a smaller contribution to productivity than anticipated this may lead to a widespread rejection of them. If so, this is unfortunate. Clearly financial incentives have a part to play in inducing extra effort and co-operation.

There is perhaps another case for the introduction of incentive bonus schemes. This flows from the enhanced power which they give to the local manager over the earnings of their subordinates. One of the frequently voiced criticisms of the centralised control of conditions of service is that local staff have no power over local rates of pay and that small details, if they do not fall into a well-defined category, have to be referred upwards for adjudication.

'The regional board to which I belong has an annual budget in excess of £80 million: but it must get permission from the Department of Health to start an officer coming from outside the service, and who is already earning more than the minimum of the appropriate scale, with one or more increments. It must also get permission from the Department for a host of trivialities: a reduction *ad absurdam* being a protracted correspondence on the subject of a course fee of half a guinea for an officer.'[4]

Incentive bonus schemes give local people more say in the level of pay of their subordinates.

We have already mentioned both the possible unwillingness of some managers to accept more responsibility and their resistance to change. A reluctance or diffidence over the implementation of incentive bonus schemes would be another straw in the same wind. 'There is indeed little enthusiasm for interim schemes from any part of the hospital service . . . to admit that an interim scheme is feasible is seen as implying slack management in the past. Departmental heads . . . feel that their scope for action might be restricted rather than extended by them . . .' The writer prophesies the gradual withering of interim schemes.[5] The reasons given for the diffidence run counter to our own suspicions of an unwillingness at least among some, to assume more responsibility. Whatever the reason we must hope diffidence does not extend to 'non-interim' bonus schemes.

A local responsibility (at least a partial one) for the level of earnings gives the manager another string to his bow. He has another means at his disposal to increase the sense of identification with the organisation's objectives.

17

Identification and Motivation

There may still be some surprise in a professional service at the suggestion that employees do not identify totally with their employer's interests. No doubt there will be less surprise after the industrial disputes in the hospital service in 1973. It is nevertheless a useful starting point from which to embark on an assessment of the contribution of this strategy to increasing productivity. Why do staff not identify with their employer?

Lupton has pointed out that identification is more likely to be with a smaller group than the organisation as a whole.

'Social science would also suggest there are limits to an individual's capacity to identify with a large organisation. There is much evidence that the behaviour of the individual is controlled more effectively by his fellows in the small group in which he works than by the formal rules and obligations of a large organisation. It is true that the organisation influences individual behaviour by working through interpersonal influence, but this is much more likely to be effective in a small organisation than in a large one comprised of many interlinked and interlocking units and sub-sub units . . .[1]

And by any definition area health authorities and district management teams are large organisations. Even below district level there will be sub-units and sub-sub units.

There is yet another possible obstacle to close identification with the objectives of the particular employing authority. Professional staff (including those we have classified as semi-professionals) may not be particularly 'loyal' to their employing organisation. Blau and Scott have described how some social welfare workers were highly critical of the standards of care in their agencies and would have willingly changed employers.[2] These workers were described as having a 'cosmopolitan' orientation to their employment. The alternative orientation was a 'local' one. Staff with this approach were identifiable by the length of time they expected to remain with their present employer and a greater acceptance of the prevailing standards of service. The basic distinction between the two groups were the reference points for comparisons with their own service. The cosmopolitan was defined as someone who chose extra-organisation sources (professional people, books, journals etc.) as the major source of intellectual and professional stimulation. The 'locals' chose sources within the employing agency (colleagues, supervisors, division head, and the director of the agency). If a cosmopolitan group exists the problems of improving efficiency through a strategy of increasing identification with the employer make its likely effect more problematic. More hopefully, Blau and Scott quote research on nurses in the United States which found that the more professional a nurse (and, therefore, had more extra-organisational reference points) the *more* likely she was to express loyalty to her work group.[3] The nurse, in short, was unlike the social welfare workers in that higher levels of professionalism did not produce a 'cosmopolitan' orientation to her employment.

An important element in a local rather than a cosmopolitan attitude to one's employment – a high level of satisfaction with the status quo – was present in a sample of state-registered nurses working in the area of the Leeds Regional Hospital Board in the late 1960s.[4] The inquiry related more to working conditions than the quality of professional service but it would not be unreasonable to assume a correlation between the two. In general, hospital nurses were more satisfied than either of the two other semi-professional groups or the community nurses which were included in the survey (*see* Table 7).

Overall the volume of criticism among our sample of nurses was slight. It was stronger among part-time staff who showed a lower level of professional commitment (measured by readership of journals, membership of Royal College of Nursing, further training etc.).[5] This tends to confirm that the Blau and Scott hypothesis about the loyalty of professionally orientated social workers may not apply to the majority of nurses in Britain. The higher levels of criticism among radiographers and physiotherapists suggests that a cosmopolitan attitude may be more prevalent among other health service professionals.

The brief digression underlies two important points for management. First that the apprenticeship system of nurse training, limited geographical mobility,[6] and the 'narrow visibility of the nurse's competence'[7] produces a local rather than a cosmopolitan

Table 8 *Attitude to employer (percentages)*

Criteria	Hospital nurses				Physiotherapists				Radiographers				District nurses and health visitors			
	Poor	All right	Good	%	Poor	All right	Good	%	Poor	All right	Good	%	Poor	All right	Good	%
1. Efficiency	7	28	64	100	4	50	46	100	19	44	37	100	14	13	73	100
2. Atmosphere of co-operation	15	26	58	100	19	22	59	100	22	25	53	100	16	24	60	100
3. Provision of the scope of work of which they felt capable	12	26	63	100	17	26	57	100	14	41	45	100	13	33	54	100
4. Opportunities for advancement	17	27	56	100	46	39	15	100	38	27	35	100	35	31	34	100

Note. Some columns do not total 100 per cent because of rounding of sub-totals.

attitude on which the manager can build more easily. Second, the strategy of improving efficiency through increased identification with an employer's interests may be more difficult with such groups as medical staff, social workers, pharmacists, engineers and physiotherapists who have received their training elsewhere and whose skills are more widely observable.

The aim of the manager must be to minimise the disparity, within these constraints, between the objectives of small groups and those of the organisation as a whole. We look at the contribution which better communications, participative management and other techniques of personnel management can make, in turn.

I BETTER COMMUNICATION SYSTEMS

The obvious starting point is the work of Professor Revans.[8] His work on hospital nurses is sufficiently well known to require only the briefest summary here. He began by examining statistics of student nurse wastage and then went on to study the attitudes of nursing staff in a number of acute hospitals. He demonstrated convincingly that there was an association between poor communications in general and low morale. For example, where there were difficulties between ward sisters and administrative staff, student nurses felt that the ward sister did little teaching and was not particularly approachable. And, perhaps most important from our point of view, hospitals with communication difficulties were less efficient. They experienced a relatively high turnover of staff, high wastage rates among student nurses and had longer-than-average lengths of stay. High turnover rates among staff, wastage of students and an unnecessarily long occupation of an expensive hospital bed clearly absorb resources. If better communications reduce the incidence of these features by increasing identification with the employer's objectives, additional resources should become available to improve the service.

There is a danger of over-reaction to this research. Communication of everything to everybody is not to be recommended either. Discrimination is required. It is not only a matter of the time taken to digest the large volume of information. Timing, too, is important. Premature consultations on the implementation of the Salmon Report led to greater anxiety and a spate of alarming rumours in some hospitals.[9]

We should be quite clear on what even a more discriminating approach to better communications can achieve too. There is considerable doubt on the efficacy of trying to raise morale, for example, through better communication. As long ago as 1957 a British psychologist felt it was time that

'the pathetic notion that you can improve communication by giving more and better information should surely be allowed to die a natural death: you will not get any reception if you are not trusted: but if relations are good, then there is a good chance that what you say will be received, and that you will get co-operation in return.'[10]

Some studies have suggested a negative relationship between more information and sympathetic attitudes towards the employer.[11] There is some doubt, too, whether more information produces greater efficiency.[12]

Since a 'free flow' of information is, generally speaking, impractical and in some cases counter-productive we have to decide in what situations different communication systems will help to increase the sense of identification with an employer and his interests. This judgement is reinforced by the obvious point that one of the purposes of hierarchical organisation, which is likely to be more important in the reformed health service, is to direct communications to the point in the structure where the information is required for decision-making. This clearly implies a restriction on the direction, content and volume of information in the interests of efficiency.

There may be occasions, however, where 'unrestricted' communication systems are helpful. There is evidence that where information passed on is not influenced by hierarchical considerations, this may be better for planning purposes.[13] An informal network is more likely to produce ideas and test those ideas rigorously. The absence of a 'senior' in the communications network lessens inhibitions about suggesting ideas. The likelihood of distortion caused by filtering of information and its presentation in a way the senior would like to hear it is reduced. All in all it produces opportunities for franker discussion. The disadvantage is the slowness with which decisions are reached.

The manager has to choose the appropriate occasion for informal communications of this type. The planning cycle, the activities of the health care planning teams, forward looks, allocation of revenue expenditure for the coming year, operational policies for new buildings, are a few examples in the non-capital field which spring to mind as possible occasions when comparatively unrestricted communicative patterns might be appropriate.

In these situations the optimal rather than a quick decision is required.

It follows that a more restricted information flow is appropriate when *a* decision is required rather than the best possible one. Extensive consultation delays the decision. Often a satisfactory decision *now* is preferable to a better decision in a week's time. In many cases immediate decisions are inescapable. Staff wanting time off to go and see an ailing relative are not helped by a system which produces decisions only after many communications with others!

The distinction between the occasions on which different information systems are appropriate is best done by a parallel. A group of people uninhibited by formal communication channels are best suited to solve a complicated jigsaw or crossword puzzle. A single decision-maker is better than a group at creating them. In the latter case one person has a framework in mind when he determines the type of puzzle or the clues. His choices are determined and co-ordinated by that framework. Others working from different starting points would make incompatible suggestions and co-ordination would be very difficult.

An intermediate stage between these two 'polar' types of communication systems are committees. What contribution can they make to better communication? Certainly the committee system in hospitals did not seem popular with the staff. 'Much of what is said about "the committee system" starts unhappily from the assumption that it is a necessary evil and at worst an irrelevance that can only impede good management.'[14] Discussions with staff in community health services produce similar responses. These assessments are probably more directed to committees of 'laymen' rather than those of professionals. It is unlikely to be the common view of the district management teams for example.

Yet communication with committees of 'laymen' can be important. One of the functions of hospital management committees, regional health boards, local health committees in the pre-reform service was to make final decisions on the allocation of resources. The staff made suggestions for change (e.g. an increase in establishment) and the boards or committees concurred, delayed or on odd occasions rejected the proposals. In this process there is intercommunication between those who control the resources and those who spend them. The latter provide information to justify their recommendations: these in turn are then in theory subject to the scrutiny of people with wider responsibilities and perspectives. The interplay of the different perspectives brings forth information which should increase appreciation of the objectives of all parties. On the one side there will be greater appreciation of the aspirations and expectations of the staff. The staff in turn should gain more insights into the pressures on the members, their concept of priorities and their aspirations for future development.

The wider perspectives of members of the area and regional health authorities are required because of the long-term implications of some changes. At these levels proposals, if approved, will set the pattern of the service for a long period: people with wider appreciative settings are required. Staff must show how their proposals fit in with the long-term and broader development of the service. At sector and district level the same pattern will be required although proposals will perhaps set the pattern for a shorter period. It is the exposure of staff to these with different 'appreciative sets' which makes committees valuable.

Properly handled, this type of interchange can increase the sense of identification with the employing body ('we' rather than 'they'). Committees, if intelligently employed, can be a useful mechanism for communication and for producing a sense of identification with the employer and a greater joint appreciation of what the major objectives should be. For our purposes, however, it is worth reminding ourselves that a committee is particularly useful if it exposes both parties to the importance of efficiency rather than adequacy: and to the extent the exchange of information produces personal dissatisfaction with the prevailing standards of efficiency.

Communications upwards are also adversely affected by too strong an identification with personal or small group interests. One of the prime needs of management either at departmental level or higher is for accurate information from the wards, primary care centres, ambulance station officers and control rooms and so on. Without good information the processes of monitoring, planning, and day-to-day decision-making are much more difficult. Where identification with an employer is strong there are fewer obstacles to this free flow of upwards information.

Yet this ideal situation is unlikely. What is communicated upwards is determined not only by formal position but personal advantage. Communication of routine information arising out of formal responsibilities should present few problems. There are few difficulties with the return of routine statistics or information on defective equipment and the staffing difficulties in departments. The problem arises when information passed on is influenced by considerations of personal advantage. The content and presentation of the information must maximise the personal advantage of the subordinate or working group, or at least ensure there is no disadvantage. After all, one's hierarchical superior is influential in one's future career ('He's the one who will write my references so I must keep in with him'). Promotion is not the only consideration. Considerations of influence and status also require that information communicated upwards must not undermine one's own position.

'Argyris reports that supervisors in an industrial setting were very selective in the information they communicated to their superiors, tending to minimise problems, to emphasise successes and to relay information detrimental to other supervisors whenever possible. . . study by Saleznick (reports) . . . manual workers were also reluctant to approach their supervisor with their problems and turned instead to their peers.'[15]

This may partially explain the reluctance of departmental heads in hospitals to volunteer for interim bonus schemes. To acknowledge the need for such a scheme is to acknowledge previous inefficiency and by implication one's own inadequacy. Filtering of information is a well-established phenomenon and a fact of life which those who wish to improve communications must take into account. It is one of the reasons, too, why senior staff are so ill-informed as to what is going on in the health service.

Clearly, the strategy of increasing identification with the employer's objectives via the medium of better communications is not without its difficulties. It is no panacea for problems of motivation and efficiency. A report on an internal communications project in the hospital service also strikes a cautious note.[16] This was a four-year action programme in which nearly forty projects were carried out by staff of the participating hospitals. The major objective was '. . . to improve hospital functioning through focusing attention on a number of goals – namely improved communication, problem-solving, and changes in the process of problem-solving. In practice, no single goal took any general precedence, although better communication . . . was the major theme.'[17] In their evaluation the authors felt that 'in terms of improving communication, the overall effects of the project seemed relatively modest . . . while in more concrete terms there seemed little change in staff turnover and absenteeism'.[18] However, they did feel there were demonstrable improvements in participating hospitals.[19]

This is not an argument against better communications in the health service. It is an argument that the limitations must be realised: that who needs what information and why must be carefully thought out: in what areas of decision-making freer communication is useful and in what areas dysfunctional, and its utility for changing perceptions, e.g. about efficiency in the desired direction, clearly assessed. Perhaps the contribution of people like Revans has been to make staff realise there is a problem; that instructions are misinterpreted, not wilfully but because of different perceptions; and that plain speaking is not all that is required (though this would sometimes help!). House journals, good relations with trade unions and staff associations, and joint discussions are useful weapons in enhancing identification provided they are used with discrimination, and their limitations are recognised.

Good communications too depend on the 'atmosphere for communication'[20] which in turn depends on 'mutual trust and respect'.[21] A technique which claims to demonstrate (and perhaps create) mutual trust and respect is participative management.

II PARTICIPATIVE MANAGEMENT

Participative management is best understood as a philosophy rather than a technique. It seeks to offer 'work which exploits individual ability and which creates for individuals opportunities to take part meaningfully in decisions about important technical and administrative questions'. [22] In more colourful terms Pantall and Elliot described some of the implications of this approach for the East Birmingham Hospitals as follows:

'... participative management, that desirable state in which management is able to draw from each according to his ability and insight, rather than his position in the hierarchical structure: that utopia . . . in which the boss realises that he might occasionally be wrong, and the subordinate realises that the boss may occasionally be right . . . participative management will not come about . . . as a result of devotional exercises or radiant bonhomie. The hospital system has to be reorganised in such a way as to encourage participation: and the very mechanics of reorganisation have to be worked out in participation . . . it means patiently sitting through meetings which crackle with atmosphere, setting the scene so that at the end of the day it begins to be seen that criticism of a service is not criticism of a person. It means ensuring that consultation is consultation and not the grudging acceptance of a well-meant *fait accompli.*'[23]

The concept is clearly more far-reaching than that of better communications though many of the techniques will be similar.

Again it is important not to over-estimate its contribution to better management. We must, for example, sound a cautionary note about the relevance of participative management to our major theme. Our main interest is the improvement in efficiency and the more frequent use of the criterion of efficiency to determine the allocation of resources. What evidence is there that participative management will help achieve these particular objectives? The answer is a rather muffled one. It is always difficult to establish cause and effect in organisational change and not all students or organisations at this stage in our knowledge are convinced about the contribution of participative management to efficiency.

Others might challenge the basic assumption of participative management that employees want to participate in decision-making. The 'hard liner' who emphasises money and compulsion as the best way to motivate employees (and others) could rightly ask for the evidence that they actually do want to do so. He could point with truth to the fairly general failure of joint consultative committees, for example, in hospitals. A survey in the late 1960s found it little used[24] and one commentator, having scrutinised the minutes of some joint consultative committees, was led to suggest they were not only ineffective but effete.[25] Intuitively, a manager might feel that at least some of the employees may want to be consulted on pay but little else: they prefer to let managers take responsibility for other things. And his intuition would have a basis in fact.[26]

We have also said there are occasions when speed of decision is preferable to the best decision if the latter takes time to emerge. If this is accepted, participative management techniques must be limited to decisions where the speed is not so essential. Otherwise there could be a decrease in efficiency. Democracy and personal growth in the health service may be a mixed blessing for the taxpayer if efficiency decreases! The spirit of participative management would not be undermined if its techniques were used to specify those decisions which require an immediate or rapid response and for which consultations would be inappropriate.

Participative management in practice
The most well-known example of this philosophy in practice in the

British health service is the experiment at the East Birmingham Hospital.[27] The research and experiment was a collaborative one between hospital and university staff. Their central concern was similar to our theme. The main objective of the manager is described thus: 'to ensure the use of resources in the best interests of patient care'. Participative management helps him to do this by finding 'ways of increasing the effectiveness of the hospital in relation to this major objective'.[28] We, of course, would be more specific and stress the improvement in the ratio of input to output and the more frequent use of the criterion of efficiency in allocative decisions.

In practice, participative management is associated with many already familiar techniques. Staff meetings, hospital journals, teach-ins, project teams and maximum delegation of authority are some obvious ones. Slightly less obvious perhaps is the association between participative management and management by objectives, job descriptions and job enlargement. The link is the philosophy behind the use of the techniques. Management by objectives and the painful process of writing job descriptions are obviously more productive in a participative climate. Job enlargement may not be so obviously linked though the ideas behind it (men ought to have more interesting work and anyway it encourages them to work harder) are similar to those of participative management.

Perhaps the most profitable way of assessing the contribution of the technique is to look again at its likely impact on decisions on the distribution of the annual increment. We have argued already that more involvement may increase identification with major organisational goals and minimise departmental ones in decision-making. If it is to do this, the approach has to be genuinely participative. Broadly speaking, there are two ways in which such discussions can be conducted. The first, all too familiar, is to 'inform' departmental heads what the allocation to the group or department is and how the increment has been distributed. The decisions, no doubt, will have been based on the estimates submitted by departments and supplemented by discussions between the individual departmental head and administrators. If this final process were done at a meeting with other departmental heads present there would be but a slight gain on the practice found in most authorities today. The slight gain would come from the opportunity for discussion and exposure to the needs of other departments which would not be so obvious in bilateral communication between departmental head and administrator. Such a procedure would not fall into the definition of participative management.

Another way of handling the same process, say at district level, is to arrange a discussion among representatives of interested parties *before* the final decisions, say on the distribution of the increment, are taken. Not only would it give those who control the resources the opportunity of hearing the views of others (which it can do on a more time-consuming individual basis), but it would also give them the opportunity to bring out problems they face – for example, is it worth increasing the establishment of physiotherapists who may not be there to recruit? It would bring into the open the question of which area, e.g. nursing, pharmacy, community or hospital services, should be given priority. Hopefully, participants would be forced to at least argue a little more in terms of the criterion of efficiency rather than adequacy.

This procedure is not without its problems: it will not produce utopia. In our example of the central dictation system a records officer was hardly likely in any circumstance to acknowledge that another department's head's needs were greater than his. Neither would the nursing officer who wanted to ensure she was fully spent on nursing salaries. And will the hospital nurse agree that community services should be given more priority at her expense? Participative management may produce greater exposure to the needs of others. It may not convince participants of their greater priority.

The second approach also raises the problems of responsibility, authority and accountability. In a truly participative situation decisions would *de facto* be taken by people represented at the meeting who to all intents and purposes would control the allocation of resources (or the increment in this example). How would they be made accountable? What could be the price of accountability? It would be anomalous if the administrator who, say, initiated the procedure was held to be accountable without comparable authority! This may be a difficulty, however, which appears more formidable in theory than it would prove to be in practice.

Another problem centres on staff groupings which would be essential to make discussions manageable. Geographical or patient groupings? And in either event where would the service departments fit in? We have commented above on the difficulty reported at East Birmingham (at least up to 1967) in producing a common purpose among departmental heads. And for a few years after 1974 would even nurses be happy with a single representative at such a meeting committing both institutional and community services? A sense of common purpose and identification with peers is a pre-requisite to effective participation. Otherwise representation and the bargaining implied by this process would prove impossible. This problem may in turn be exacerbated among nursing staff by the traditional authority accorded to their seniors and consequently a reluctance on the part of some staff to be drawn into a participative management system.

However, the second approach to making decisions on the allocation of resources (which is much nearer the participative model than what usually happens at the moment) is more likely to *change* the perceptions of staff. And we are agreed that perceptions about resources, their use and allocation, have to be changed to provide greater efficiency. It will change appreciations only if the pre-requisite of commitment to this style of management is present. The sad history of joint consultation machinery in the hospital service is proof of that.

The key to success is not only commitment to the philosophy, however, but a realistic assessment of its potential, and an understanding of what type of decision for which extensive consultations are suited. Commitment is vital, particularly on the part of senior managers and departmental heads. Without their commitment the impetus and drive would be lacking. It is appropriate to leave the final assessment to the East Birmingham researchers.

'Participative management seems to us in the end to mean:
1. A recognition that main managerial decisions have to be made at the centre.
2. A genuine and deeply felt intent to help the task of central decision-making by pushing as much discretion as possible outwards, through the organisation.
3. A system which does not grudgingly permit, but actively encourages the front line of staff to bring their experience and knowledge into the service of management.'[29]

III PERSONNEL MANAGEMENT

Personnel managers would rightly object to any implication that their responsibilities were confined to reducing the importance of identification with groups or sub-groups. Their responsibilities are broader. However, in this section we do concentrate on the rather disparate techniques available to increase the identification of the employee with the interests of the wider concern. Within this narrow framework it is the impact of supervisory styles which demands most of our attention. The partial assessment of the contribution of personnel management is explained by the major theme of the book – how to increase efficiency – and of this chapter – higher productivity from greater identification with the employer's major objectives.

(a) Pride of performance

All employees have a need for self-expression and self-fulfilment though its importance may differ between different types of staff. We are surer of its importance for professional and managerial staff (partly perhaps because there is a greater chance of their needs being met). Personnel policies which attempt to organise work routines and job specifications to meet these needs may result in greater job satisfaction and a stronger identification with the employer's interests. Rewards can be tied to jobs well done and to the quality of work rather than sheer output as with most incentive schemes. This is the rationale for 'zero defects' and 'pride of performance' campaigns. Such techniques are important in American hospitals where perhaps the need to increase productivity is given greater priority.[30]

(b) Job dissatisfaction and staff welfare schemes

Job enlargement aims to provide satisfaction and thereby increase identification. So do many other welfare schemes. But an important objective of personnel management is to remove causes of job dissatisfaction.

The causes of dissatisfaction are not the obverse of sources of satisfaction. While the latter include recognition for achievement, the value of work itself, personal growth and responsibility at work, the sources of dissatisfaction are of a slightly different order. They include company policy administration, relationship with supervisors and other factors focusing on conditions of service.[31] We shall follow Herzberg and call the causes of job dissatisfaction 'hygienic factors'.

Clearly many staff welfare policies have the twin aim of promoting satisfaction and removing causes of dissatisfaction. We shall look primarily at their contribution to the latter. One immediate objection has to be met. The conditions of employment of most staff are negotiated centrally. There may thus be little scope for the manager in the service to do much himself to remove sources of dissatisfaction. Before reform this was a more justifiable feeling among hospital service personnel than those in local authorities.

Yet there are examples in the health service of great efforts to remove sources of dissatisfaction. An excellent illustration is the experiment at the Hendon Group Hospital Management Committee. This particular scheme is very apposite, since it was in the hospital service before 1974 that there was less scope for local initiative to remove dissatisfactions centred on conditions of service. We do not describe the introduction of the scheme here – readers are referred to the journals for this.[32] Our interest is the opportunities available to health staff (not merely personnel officers) to combat causes of job dissatisfaction.

An important element in the scheme was the collection of information. For example, terminal interviews with all staff who were leaving were conducted.[33] For one who suffered from returns indicating 'personal reasons' were the cause of departure in 99·9 per cent of cases, information from interviews is an obvious improvement. This was supplemented by an 'opinion survey' of all grades of other staff. They were to be asked questions on working conditions, general problems affecting their jobs, career prospects in the group and ways of improving matters. An attack on the causes of discontent which can lead to high turnover rates must be well informed.

There was sufficient discretion for local initiatives. Accommodation for staff was one such area. Accommodation (which obviously is a 'hygienic factor') was felt to be a problem in the recruitment rather than retention of staff. 'This (problem) has been eased considerably by the department arranging accommodation for members of the staff, particularly those moving to the area from the provinces. It is hoped to extend this service by providing a staff hostel.'[34]

Another example was the initiation of sick visiting of all employees who had been ill for more than a month. The official rationale behind this move was 'to maintain interest at a time when morale is usually low and to assist with any domestic problems'.[35] Absences for sickness are of course influenced by social and psychological factors. An expression of personal concern coupled with offers of practical help might combat some of these factors.

(c) The quality of supervision

A critical area in personnel management is supervisory styles. Poor supervision is directly linked, for example, with staff turnover.[36] It is linked too with higher rates of absenteeism and low productivity. All are crucial constraints in any drive to increase efficiency. They have real costs which absorb unnecessary resources.

Improvements in this area of personnel management are more important than more strenuous attempts to recruit staff. At Hendon it was realised that expensive recruitment campaigns were putting the cart before the horse. 'A recruiting officer could only try to keep up with the pace of staff wastage, whereas the emphasis should be on reducing wastage and thus relieving the burden of recruitment.'[37]

The human relations school who particularly stress the importance of supervision in management, starts from the premise that most employees want to work, to express themselves and be recognised for achievement.[38] The task of the manager and supervisor is to harness these drives and to use the group loyalties, recognised as important since the famous Hawthorne experiments, to improve performance.

Popularly, the argument leads to a widespread feeling that democratic and participative management styles are essential. Certain authoritarian styles are considered counter-productive. Close supervision of the employee's work is one ('Let's make sure you've made the beds correctly nurse'). Others include demonstrating one's belief in strictness rather than taking a relaxed view of relations with subordinates (the old dragon syndrome); an approach which workers consider to be unfriendly and unfavourable ('You can't really trust them to do jobs properly'); issuing instructions which are felt to be less than clear; and when supervisors are felt to stick too closely to rules and be reluctant to make exceptions ('She's swallowed the rule book').[39]

The styles or traits are unhelpful because the supervisor needs full co-operation to improve on a minimum level of output. Formal authority is insufficient to motivate subordinates. Certainly it gives superiors the right to assign jobs and responsibilities; and even select his own subordinates in some cases. Yet in itself formal authority is of little value in increasing productivity. Ordering a cleaner to work harder or to accept a change in working practice is hardly likely to produce a sustained and worthwhile result.

The more effective supervisors acquire informal authority necessary to motivate subordinates above minimal or insufficient levels of output. They do this by providing services which build up a network of obligations. An example which immediately springs to mind is the supervisor who uses his power to ignore the rules, gets equipment repaired quickly (e.g. the bedpan steriliser!), arranges off-duty to suit the nurse who wants to see her boyfriend, fights for a new theatre changing room for men, and resists impossible demands on radiography, physiotherapy, medical laboratories and district nurses. Rendering these kinds of service creates obligations, and subordinates who are obliged to their supervisor for benefits received will feel they should reciprocate by complying with his requests and special demands.[40] An authoritarian approach has been found to be less effective in building up these feelings of obligations and loyalty to the supervisor. And there is evidence to suggest that the base of obligations and loyalty is a pre-requisite for extra effort.[41]

If supervisors in the health service can develop this informal authority and loyalty to themselves, then it is their objectives which become the crucial ones. Their efforts must be directed to the objectives which other members of the organisation have agreed are paramount. One of these major objectives must be increased efficiency.

So far we have talked primarily of the impact of supervisory styles on the performance of manual workers. The picture *vis-à-vis* professional staff is less clear. Research in the United States has suggested that the relationship between the democratic supervision of social workers and effort was a little more complex.[42]

Authoritarian practices did have a negative impact. They were associated, for example, with an unwillingness to take initiatives, frequent consultations with supervisors and a larger proportion of time in group meetings taken up with directives.[43] This description seems very close to the relationships which exist in many parts of the health service today. In Blau and Scott's study, however, these features of supervisory style did not result in inferior productivity: it was more likely to produce less job satisfaction.[44] If this holds true for health service personnel in Britain then factors other than the style of supervision are important in enhancing productivity. Interestingly, the authors of the Hendon scheme had assumed an association between high staff turnover and the quality of supervision. They say in passing that this was 'not subsequently borne out by more detailed investigation'.[45] This observation seems to refer to all types of staff.

The suggestion that there would be few gains among professional workers in terms of higher productivity or lower turnover rates is supported by the relatively modest improvements produced by the hospital internal communications project. It might of course be true that the poor communications/authoritarian supervisory style syndrome has other ill effects and therefore improvements in supervision would still be profitable.

Superficially it would seem that the answer to our problem of increasing identification with the employer's interests, at least as far as manual workers are concerned, lies in the training of supervisors. Properly trained they will be better able to promote job satisfaction and minimise dissatisfaction. Even among professional workers there may also be gains.

It is advisable to counsel against unrealistic expectations. First, because it hardly seems likely that some jobs can ever be really satisfying. Disbelievers only have to look at the evidence of what proportion of workers would choose the same occupations again given the choice.[46] Improving the quality of supervision, the use of other techniques like job enlargement and job rotation will give more satisfaction or reduce the levels of dissatisfaction. But for most manual workers the level of job satisfaction must remain pretty low. 'Motivating' them will be a permanent managerial problem. Lupton takes this point further. In talking about the likely impact of incentive schemes on restriction of output he asks 'whether it would be best to leave the group restricting output . . . Since it would appear unaided they have found ways to satisfy their needs by using their power to control the job, which management had not built into the formal organisation.'[47]

Second, it is possible to become so involved with improving relationships within the organisation, causes of job dissatisfaction and seeking to increase satisfaction, that the job itself gets short shrift. It is important to realise the limits placed on the success of these policies and the dangers of too much emphasis on staff needs at the expense perhaps of service to patients.

Third, there are limits to the change which can be wrought by training schemes. People with authoritarian personalities are not going to change their spots overnight, if ever. A human relations approach to supervision without ideological commitment may be worse than a consistently authoritarian one. Training can help the committed to be more effective: it might help the waverer. It is this modest level of change to which one aspires with existing personnel.

Having sounded a note of caution it is obvious that if the quality of supervision can be improved even slightly it is a worthwhile objective. A 2 per cent increase in productivity among a staff complement of 500 produces the equivalent of ten more staff. What we know of the low level of productivity among hospital staff suggests this level of improvement can be maintained for many years to come. The position in community services is less clear though no doubt there is scope for more intensive use of scarce skills.

What of professional staff? We need to be more positive about the features of supervisory styles which will produce a response from them. One is consistency of behaviour. Blau and Scott[48] found that this feature in supervision, measured by the consistency with which the subordinates evaluated the supervisor's performance on seven different aspects of behaviour, was directly related to loyalty. The more consistent the supervisor the more loyal were the subordinates. There was also a suggestion that a self-confident supervisor who was strict received more loyalty than one who was lenient: the obverse obtained with a supervisor who was unsure.

This serves to warn us that a supervisory style independent of the personality of the supervisor and staff to be supervised is ineffective and possibly counter-productive. A self-confident authoritarian ward sister or health visitor – if these findings apply to her – who adopts a lenient approach to staff because that seems nearer the democratic mode of supervision, would be doing herself a disservice.

Another feature of supervisory styles which Blau and Scott found to be linked with greater loyalty among subordinates was the hierarchical independence of the supervisor from his chief. The greater the degree of independence the greater the loyalty among subordinates.[49]

Hierarchical independence was measured by the difference in the approach of the supervisor and his or her superior. It was associated with fewer expressions of loyalty to the supervisor's boss. Independence had to be linked of course with sufficient autonomy to satisfy subordinates. The loyalty of subordinates was in turn a source of social support for the independent supervisors for whom there was little peer group support.

We do not know whether loyalty of subordinates to supervisors in the British Health Service would be increased by displays of hierarchical independence. In the absence of substantive evidence, however, we can take it as a working hypothesis. We then have to ask whether conditions in the health service are conducive to hierarchical independence of supervisors. It would seem to be more likely for some than for others. For example, non-nursing departmental heads might find it easier to be independent, particularly if there was no medical head of the department. This may be true even where there are medical heads of a department. One was always struck by the sturdy independence of the chief laboratory technician who seemed equally independent of pathologist and administrator: or even the biochemist in the same laboratory! The pharmacist has no obvious senior and this makes independence of the administrator much easier and acceptable. In the case of nurses it would be interesting to know to what extent, if any, the Salmon and Mayston schemes have reduced the sturdy independence of sisters, or whether it is still possible to be as hierarchically independent in the more clearly defined and bureaucratic system of management as it was before. It is possible that the community nurse attached to a practice may be relatively independent of the area nursing officer.

These were the two factors which Blau and Scott found to be most important in developing group solidarity among social workers. A third was 'emotional detachment', which subsumed the ability to retain one's temper.[50] Perhaps, too, the intensely formal 'Mr Smith' for the most junior staff can find a justification in organisational theory!

The differences between various groups of staff and supervisors underlines the need for a discriminating and flexible approach to theories of supervision. Blanket remedies whether they be 'more and better communication', 'participative management', 'the need for more/better supervision', are not the answer. With manual workers we can be more confident, for example, of the beneficial impact of democratic styles. A study of ten American acute general hospitals indicated that the ability to handle people became more important the 'lower' down the hierarchy one went.[51] Generally speaking leadership patterns should not merely reflect theory. They should also reflect the personalities of the managers, their subordinates, and the reality of the situation on the ground.[52]

We can develop this argument for flexibility of response a little further. Schatz[53] writes of a company introducing a formal employee evaluation by supervisors which might with profit be followed more often in the health service. It was specified that the evaluation, however, was to cover not only the employee's 'strengths and interests' but his weaknesses. The supervisor was also evaluated partly on whether he included points of criticism in his report as well as favourable ones.

Two things might follow from this kind of assessment. First, the possibility of some readjustment of work, transfer or training to take advantage of the good points and minimise the effects of the bad. It allows jobs to be built round employees' strengths and reduces the emphasis on trying to strengthen their weaknesses. There is obvious scope for such 'job building' in many departments in the health service, particularly after integration. Such an exercise might reduce dissatisfaction with hygienic factors as well as promote more job satisfaction.

A second implication is that the supervisor acknowledges the employee's weaknesses and can try to compensate for them. A good illustration of this kind of thinking is found in an article by a geriatrician in *The Hospital*.[54]

He argues: '. . . the physicians must make the most of poor material'. Standards of performance can be raised by the use of applied psychology to avoid stresses and strains which disturb mental attitudes and lower efficiency'. Only those proficient in applied psychology may feel sufficiently confident to make such a claim, although most supervisors would try to avoid stressful situations and strain. More specifically, Howell mentions discussions or conferences over routines for recurrent problems and visits to other units as examples of how the consultant can help the nursing staff. Such techniques are clearly not beyond the ken of most managers. If we accept Howell's analysis it may be inevitable that staff will be hired with ability below the 'norm desirable': and that consequently the manager must recognise that too high expectations of them and the unexpected cause strain. Improved performance follows efforts to minimise these strains.

(d) Recruitment and training

There are other ways to combat job dissatisfaction, promote satisfaction and develop greater identification with the objectives of the organisation. Recruitment and training policies also help. A story from the Hendon scheme is almost in itself sufficient to make the case for more systematic attention to recruitment. 'Geographically at Edgware General Hospital departments are scattered and difficult to find. Many intending applicants arrived at the main gate, perhaps feeling a little nervous, got lost in the corridors of the hospital and never arrived at the point of interview and consequently a percentage of the potentially available labour was lost.'[55] One can only admire the authors for such a frank admission. Even without a personnel officer there is obviously something the manager can clearly do to improve recruitment! And this also applies to selection procedures.

It is obvious that the suitability of staff for the job is a constraint on the improvements that can be expected from better man (and woman) management. There are limits to the compensation one can make for ineffective performance; or for the dissatisfactions over hygienic factors because of misunderstandings at the time of appointment; or for an authoritarian domestic forewoman, etc. If a suitable person is employed in the first place then we can expect better results. It is not merely a matter of selecting the most suitable person. An intelligent approach to man management may identify groups who might fit better into the particular health service environment. For example, at the Hendon it was found that labour turnover could be reduced by recruiting porters from the age group of forty-five plus as this was the age group which exhibited the greatest stability in employment.[56]

It may also be argued that efficient selection needs expertise, which many do not have. This applies even to the preparation of the job specifications (job descriptions with the qualities the incumbent requires) which should precede shortlisting and interviews. It is commonly accepted that eliciting information in a twenty-minute interview from often inarticulate people requires special skills. Yet in the absence of a personnel officer to supply these skills staff can do something to improve their own selection techniques. (Indeed a recognition that others have the skills is an advance for some!)

It is training which is the watchword in the health service today. The reform of the service is being prepared at the time of writing amid a welter of integration courses for first-, middle- and top-line managers. The use of this strategy to improve the sense of identification depends on availability of suitable courses and willingness of staff to go, as well as the attitude of senior management. There are things the first-line and middle manager can do for themselves, however. They can legitimately ask for information on the impact of training, and try to encourage the ex-trainee to use his new-found expertise.

There are few doubts (if any) about the value of induction courses. It is during early weeks of employment when emotional stress is at its peak that the decision to leave is often taken. Help and support, preferably in the form of a brief but systematic introduction, produces dividends if the new employee can be helped over what has been called the induction crisis.

Even if there are no formal provisions (which is inexcusable) for induction training, heads of departments or sections can do much to help new employees over this difficult period. The employee needs to know much about conditions of service, location of staff rooms and canteens and other departments, who does what and where. Sensibility to the need for this kind of information is not beyond the scope of managers. An introduction to the working procedures within the department or area is required even where there is formal induction training. This is particularly necessary for those with little or no previous experience of the health services and without a specific skill to offer. On-the-job training on a planned systematic basis falls too within the province of the manager. What can be done is demonstrated by some enterprising managers who have ensured cleaners, for example, can be taught how to handle cleaning equipment, economy of movement, noise control and control of infection among other things.[57]

A little later in the induction process Cuming also commends the use of settling-in interviews. These he feels are best conducted three or four weeks after the new employee has commenced work. These present a structured opportunity 'to discuss any difficulties or problems experienced with their new jobs or working conditions, before it becomes too late to do anything constructive about them'.[58]

Induction training is doubly relevant to our theme. Not only does it reduce labour turnover, which reduces the real costs in obtaining and inducting (haphazardly) new staff, but it also helps to remove causes of dissatisfaction and thus promotes identification with the objectives of the employer. Clearly managers, and not just the specialists, have an important role in this process. This is not confined to compensating for the lack of formal arrangements. Even where they exist there is a need to complement them. Whether this happens depends on the managers' awareness of the importance of this induction period, and their ability to raise their eyes beyond the everyday routines which are given precedence over more strategic concerns. To do so will probably give them a bigger return on the time invested than some of those routine everyday demands on their time.

Another species of training is the post-professional variety. Refresher courses for medical staff, nursing staff, professional and technical staff, records officers, engineers, etc. are essential to keep staff abreast of current developments. We mention this type of training only in passing because the capacity of the manager to compensate for its absence is more limited. In its absence, say for nursing staff returning after a number of years away from the service, the manager will do well to remember the newcomer's probable feelings of inadequacy. Competent managers will try to offset these feelings within the limits of their ability to boost the confidence and self-esteem of the returned prodigal.

The largest 'growth point' is, however, management training. At the time of writing there are integration courses for first-, middle- and top-line managers in the health service. These supplement existing management training schemes. Unfortunately there is little hard evidence of how effective these courses are! Evaluation is difficult and at this stage we must reserve judgement.

One of the problems which has to be overcome is the perception of staff who do not see themselves as managers. This is not to say they do not have managerial responsibilities. It is rather that such responsibilities are seen as peripheral to their 'real' job. A survey conducted among thirty-five members of multidisciplinary first-line and middle-level hospital managers suggested that management responsibilities were carried out unconsciously and were seens as a residual function.[59] This fits with a distinct impression the author had of a first-line management course of nurses. At the end of the course one felt that the nurses had seen management techniques as useful because they would enable them to get through their management chores (often presented as boring clerical work) quicker and thus allow them to get back to their real job – nursing the patient.[60] Williams argues that if his evidence too is supported by general experience, courses on management techniques are less productive than an alternative strategy of awakening professional staff to their management responsibilities in the first place. He suggests that the simple expedient of job analysis questionnaires can assist in the process of increasing appreciation of one's job.[61] This suggests managers (if *they* have the appreciation!) *can* help their junior staff to understand more clearly what their job is all about.

IV THE STRATEGY OF ADAPTATION

Much of the material relevant to Galbraith's fourth organisational inducement has been included in the long section on identification. Perhaps the key element, which provides a slightly different focus to that used in the previous section is the question of delegation. Without some elbow room for initiative in the lower echelons, this particular need cannot be met and a strategy of motivating the employee would have to exclude this option.

The service can more easily offer this inducement in a 'participative management' system than its converse. In such a system the employee would have a greater opportunity to press his own objectives for acceptance by others. To the extent that participative management implies maximum delegation of decision-making with the requisite minimum authority this will be doubly so. In a system which encourages initiative (as maximum delegation must do), the need for adaptation can be more readily met.

The case for maximum delegation is a much broader one than meeting the factor of adaptation. It rests on arguments about enhanced motivation of the worker and the freeing of the more senior from routine work, among other things. But without a clearer set of operational objectives, identification of key areas for action and acceptance of the 'right' criterion for decisions (efficiency), the cry of 'more delegation' has little more merit than other slogans for better management so often heard in the service. The personnel to whom the decisions are delegated must march in the right direction.

The strategy of increasing motivation by meeting employees' adaptive needs carries with it very far-reaching implications. Not only is there the rather tiresome discussion of whether or not one can also delegate commensurate responsibility (it is agreed one cannot). There is also the question of authority. Jaques points out that to make a manager accountable he must have the authority necessary to discharge his responsibilities and this implies, for example, an effective veto over staff appointments, as well as the right to have inefficient employees removed.[62]

V   CONCLUSION

Many important features of personnel management have been ignored or mentioned here very briefly. This was inevitable given our frame of reference. We have looked at personnel management to see in what ways it might further the objective of increasing efficiency. In doing so we have placed much stress on the importance of increased identification with the employer's interests.

It must be remembered that other features of organisational life 'influence' the decision-maker to act in the way perceived to be in the best interests of the organisation. Simon categorises these influences as divisions of work, standard practices, downward transmission of decisions by the establishment of authority and influence, channels of communication and training.[63] Training 'injects into the very nervous system of the organisation's members the criteria of decision that the organisation wishes to employ. The organisation member acquires knowledge, skill and identifications or loyalties that enable him to make decisions, by himself, as the organisation would like him to decide.' [64]

We have discussed only some of these techniques.

Our bird's-eye view of personnel techniques has, however, indicated some of the ways in which they may contribute to increased efficiency. The lessons, too, are clear. They will not be successful if adopted uncritically or without discrimination: they must be adapted to local situations. Unrealistic expectations of the contribution such techniques can make to increased efficiency are also to be avoided. The drive for more democratic management, for example, owes something to value judgements about how people *should* be treated; whether this produces greater efficiency is another question. We have assumed for the most part that it does.

Efficient man management is not an end in itself. Its place in the scheme of things is to produce a surplus of resources which can be then reinvested to produce a better service. The two are not always easy bedfellows. For example the implication that the level of funds allocated in the past to a department are *not* sacrosanct is likely to produce considerable heart-searching. An increase in loyalty to the supervisor may lead to increased productivity among members: but this loyalty might then prove to be a bigger obstacle to a transfer of funds because of the possible loss of power, discretion and status. Yet without such a diversion of funds the benefits of better staff management would be partly dissipated. Where the two conflict, priority must be given to considerations of efficiency. Otherwise the staff's desire for development and a level of service much nearer their own conception of adequacy will not be met.

18

The Manager and the Patient

So far the book has resembled Hamlet without the Prince of Denmark. Most of the people to whom this book is addressed perceive their function as patient-centred. Their primary purpose is to help the patient who so far has been mentioned only briefly. Now it is time to remedy this omission.

We need first to demonstrate how this topic fits into a book which has hitherto concentrated on the efficient use of resources. Clearly staff/patient relationships are an important element (some would say the only important one) in the quality of service to the consumer. Some would feel (including the author) that the quality of these relationships are guaranteed more by training and professional ethics than by the question of resources.

There are three ways in which the subject is important for our theme of the more efficient use of resources. The first relates to the ultimate objective of the Service. Efficient use of resources is not an end in itself. Its rationale is the freeing of resources to improve services to the patient. This chapter is required to remind us of this fact.

Second, there *is* an association between resources and relationships. Some would argue that the absence of resources, e.g. in the psychiatric and geriatric services, are directly related to the scandals that have surfaced in the last few years. Some would also feel there was a conflict between efficiency and good staff/patient relationships, particularly when the latter were felt to be dependent on more time being available to foster them. It is important to be clear about the relationship between resources and the quality of care.

Third, in this aspect of care, few staff would deny the importance of their individual contribution. Consequently, if they were convinced that there were areas in which the relationship might be improved, it might seem more directly related to their own contribution than did the discussions about the more efficient use of resources. Though this is a conclusion we would not accept, it

166

helps to underline the responsibility of managers in the Service and the contribution which they can make.

These are the ways in which the subject is relevant to our theme. There is, however, an overriding reason why it should be discussed fully here. In future, it is an area of management which will increasingly attract the attention of those in the service.

There may be some who will be surprised at this assertion. They feel that there are in reality very few problems of staff/patient relationships which therefore hardly merit the attention they receive in this chapter. Those who share this point of view may well feel that patients' interests are well protected by the professional ethics of those who care for them. Certainly one group – the nurses – see themselves as the major spokesmen for the patients in the new service. 'The biggest criticism of the government's plans is that it lacks the chance of full consumer participation. Nurses are better placed than any single group to speak on behalf of the patients. They know their needs at night in the home and in the out-patient clinics.'[1] So often every action taken by the doctor or nurse is said to be 'in the best interests of the patient'.

Not all reject the notion that there is a conflict of interest which makes for problems in staff/patient relationships. 'However, if . . . the hospital is run for staff as much as for patients there is a risk that if it is run by staff it may be run excessively for the staff.'[2]

This is the view of someone inside the service and not one of the 'uninformed' from the outside world. This is not to say that health services run by staff *are* run with too little regard for the interests of patients. The quotation merely acknowledges that it is a possibility, and this admission carries with it the implication that there is a potential conflict of interests between provider and consumer.

The past decade has taught us that professional ethics alone will not ensure that the balance will always be tilted in favour of patients' interests. If they have done nothing else, the scandals in the long-stay institutions enable us to make this judgement with confidence. It is sobering to record the 'highlights' of these exposés. Barbara Robb's efforts in *Sans Everything*[3] in 1967 was quickly followed by official reports on Ely[4] (1969), Farleigh[5] (1971) and Whittingham[6] (1972) hospitals. There is no need to recount the stories themselves here. It is sufficient to note that in the last three reports there was official confirmation of the appalling conditions and generally poor services which led in some isolated instances to brutality and downright dishonesty. It has become harder, too to argue that these events are isolated and there is no general problem of relationships between staff and patients at least in long-stay hospitals. The annual reports of the hospital advisory service indeed suggest that the problem persists in a number of hospitals.[7] In a description of the geriatric services in 1971 the Director refers to what he calls the 'waiting syndrome' which the teams still found on many wards. On these wards patients were often woken early and spent most of the day waiting for meals or bedpan rounds. The same report highlights the problem of getting staff to see that the patients' interests are being neglected. While some respond with pride at the speed with which patients adjust to hospital routines, the relatives 'are often aghast at the obvious loss of individuality and interest in life'.[8]

There is other evidence of a more general and theoretical kind. Goffman, for example, has written much on the effects of hospitals, particularly psychiatric ones, on the patient. In many long-stay institutions he sees patient management facilitated by 'routine . . . dictated not by medical considerations, but by other factors, notably rules . . . that have emerged in an institution for the comfort and convenience of staff'.[9] Patients have to be 'deceived' about certain procedures to give the impression of them being medically necessary to get them to accept these rules.[10]

Nor is the problem confined to long-stay institutions. In the 1960s there was considerable criticism of the maternity services.[11] Orthopaedics may also be a specialty which attracts a disproportionate amount of criticism from consumers.[12] Departments of paediatrics have come in for their share of criticism too. A large part of these criticisms concerned relationships between staff and patients. Community services, except for complaints about paucity of their provision, seemed to come through relatively unscathed.

The problem must not be overstated. There is, for example, the evidence of widespread approval of the health service.[13] Although the PEP report refers to a period of time when the service was in its infancy, subsequent reports have commented on the widespread satisfaction expressed, for example, by hospital patients. In a study of an acute hospital in Manchester, the author, with four other zealous trainees, found many patients unwilling to criticise anything.[14] This is the experience of others. In Scotland, Vera Carstairs found that in general hospitals the vast majority of in- and out-patients were very satisfied with the service. In mental hospitals too, the majority were either very or fairly satisfied with the service.[15] Ann Cartwright, in an earlier study, commented critically on a similarly large expression of satisfaction with the status quo. 'But the most disturbing bequest from earlier traditions of philanthropy is the acceptance by the patients, public and medical and nursing professions of the poor, outmoded conditions in many hospitals today.'[16]

Indeed, some would argue that there has been too much attention paid to the interests of patients at the expense of staff. 'Anyone who has visited hospitals in Britain and other countries in the last twenty years must be struck by the greater emphasis on patients' comfort and privacy in the British hospital. . . .' Comfort at times seems to have taken precedence over efficiency and safety.[17] Examples of this over-indulgence are the angle-poise lamp, which is good for reading but not medical examinations, and the appearance of the flower room 'in ward design before the extra laboratory space needed for precise measurement on which safety depends'.[18] Dr Ellis is acknowledging a conflict of interest – in this case between comfort and safety – and the balance has swung too much in favour of the former. He would see the problem rather differently – how to redress the balance in favour of staff'. (In favour of staff because they represent the forces of safety in diagnosis and treatment.)

All this suggests that there may be problems now in reaching a satisfactory balance between patient and staff interests in a minority of cases. In future it may be a much more problematic area of management because of the social revolution of which we hear so much. Better education, housing, higher material standards go along with higher expectations which will probably make the consumer more, rather than less, sensitive to indifferent personal service. The greater willingness of younger people to criticise compared with their elders suggests that this change may be already on the way.[19]

It is clear that patient/staff relationships will be a sensitive area in the integrated health service; that there is, at least on occasions, a conflict of interest between staff and patient; and that we cannot rely exclusively on the professional ethics of the practitioner to strike a fair balance between the two. The management problem will be to identify these areas where interests conflict and ensure a fair (and perhaps changing) balance is maintained.

THE CONFLICT OF INTERESTS

It is essential to establish in what areas there is a potential clash of interests. Since we are arguing for a patient-centred service we approach this question from the consumer's standpoint. The main reason the patient seeks aid from the health services is to remedy some real or imagined ill-health. In doing so, the patient gives the practitioner authority to do what he will to make him well again. Goffman points out that this gives the practitioner the same type of authority as one gives the garage mechanic to rectify a fault in the car. It is a service contract and does not give the practitioner the authority to do anything more than what is required to treat the illness.[20] While the practitioner is doing this he has the requisite authority: there is no major clash of interests.[21]

The clash of interests is more likely to arise in those areas of service not covered by the service agreement. And these become more important where patients seek service because they are in need of care rather than medical treatment. Non-medical areas where conflicts of interest occur range from multisex wards which increase productivity but reduce privacy; arrangements for the visiting of patients, food, heating, routines in the wards, to arrangements for discharge. In the community, visiting of patients by general practitioners seems to be another area for a potential clash of interest. In both sectors medical information to the patient probably falls into this category.

An argument that there will be more attention paid to achieving a fair balance between staff and patients' interests is not an argument for the total precedence of patient interests. Where there is a conflict, a balance has to be struck. A situation in which too much precedence was given to patients' comforts (e.g. the flower room) may not be in the medical interests of those same patients! Or a situation may become intolerable for staff who have legitimate interests too which must be considered.

THE ORGANISATIONAL EQUILIBRIUM AND THE PATIENT'S CONTRIBUTION

The concept of organisational equilibrium helps us to understand this balance a little more. Herbert Simon's concept of the organisation equilibrium envisages a three-part contribution. In addition to the customer and staff, there is the contribution of the entrepreneur.[22] In the National Health Service the Department itself, the new authorities and senior managers, approximate to this third group.

All three groups 'accept organisational membership when their activity in the organisation contributes, directly or indirectly, to their own personal goals'.[23] These goals cannot be met in their entirety. An equilibrium between the goals of the participants has to be reached.

'The members of an organisation, then, contribute to the organisation in return for inducements that the organisation offers them. The contributions of one group are the sources of the inducements that the organisation offers others. If the sum of the contributions is sufficient, in quantity and kind, to supply the necessary quantity and kinds of inducements, the organisation survives and grows; otherwise it shrinks and ultimately disappears unless an equilibrium is reached'.[24]

Signs of disequilibrium in the context of British health services would be less dramatic: resignations of members and staff are more likely manifestations. Complaints from patients, their relatives or consumer organisations would increase.

The point at which an equilibrium is reached is not fixed. It clearly changes over time. One only has to make a superficial comparison of hospital life to appreciate this point. It is not only changing in relation to patients' interests; the balance between the entrepreneurs and staff has been and will continue to be changed, too.

The management of the organisational equilibrium is facilitated by another factor – the willingness of staff, patients and controllers to accept rules, decisions and policies when they do not further their own objectives but do not obviously conflict with them either. This phenomenon in a slightly more restricted context has been referred to as the 'zone of acceptance'.[25] Decisions will be acted upon not only if they are consistent with the participant's own objectives but also when they do not seem particularly relevant or are not in conflict with them.

The precise balance which is struck varies from place to place, and even within units. At Whittingham, for example, the committee of inquiry remarked on the difference between the admission wards and special units where the patients 'seem much like those in any other modern hospital environment' and the long-stay patients who 'show every sign of an absence of medical treatment and rehabilitation'.[26] The needs of the latter were not given the precedence given to those of the former; an illustration of a different balance between the interests of staff, patients and controllers even within an institution. No doubt there are similar differences between the different areas under the control of the same local health authority.

THE ORGANISATIONAL EQUILIBRIUM AND THE
MANAGER'S PROBLEM

The equilibrium presents two kinds of management problem. First, when there is an obvious state of disequilibrium, manifesting itself, for example, in an increasing volume of complaints from patients, their relatives or consumer organisations about, say, a particular unit, clinic or practice, or more rapid staff turnover. The 'new broom' may produce such a situation. A 'with-it' obstetrician coming into a straight-laced maternity unit in the early 1960s, insisting on a modernisation programme which included the right of fathers if they so requested to be present at the birth of their child, may produce a difficult situation. Some long-standing members of the department may not like it, morale would sag and perhaps some staff would leave. A new psychiatrist taking over a neglected area in mental subnormality is a parallel example. In these cases the management task is not to restore the status quo. It is rather to facilitate the change by appropriate recruitment, retraining and counselling.

Second, there is the situation where there is an equilibrium of sorts but it is manifestly unfair. Whittingham before 'the *affaire*' surfaced is a good example. A more common example may be what we can call the 'humanitarian/authoritarian situation'. In wards, units, or clinics where this situation obtains staff are personally very kind and concerned. However, patients are rigidly controlled. In one geriatric hospital, in the writer's experience, patients were always kept clean and comfortable; nurses always had a kind word for them. Patients, however, were expected to stay in bed until fairly late in the morning until much of the cleaning work was done. The floors were spotless and terrifyingly shiny! Patients were encouraged to conform by a number of informal rules, for example, about the time spectacles became available.

These situations may be less frequent now but this is not the issue here. It is the general description of a possible situation. It may be asked in what sense is there a management problem if an equilibrium has been reached? There are two ways in which it is a management problem. First it is an insecure situation based partly on the unwillingness (and inability) of certain patients to complain. As patients become more willing to complain – or visitors or pressure groups on their behalf do so – these situations may present crises of a considerable magnitude if not tackled in good time. Second, they are problems, even if these crises are unlikely, because to some parties to the equilibrium they are unfair.

An important element in both kinds of management problem in achieving a satisfactory balance of interests is an accurate appreciation of the patient's needs. Since patients are in a weak bargaining position, staff have to compensate for them to ensure their interests are adequately considered. It is wrong to see patients as a homogeneous group with common needs. There is an infinite variety of patients and staff must appreciate their differences if relationships are to be well managed.

The first and most obvious difference is the patient's clinical condition. Seriously ill and long-stay patients have one thing in common – a great dependence on staff. Such patients are unlikely to complain or use more indirect methods to show their unhappiness with particular rules. In a long-stay hospital patients will not usually jeopardise their future relationship with staff to obtain more freedom of action. In most cases the humanity of staff clearly compensates for any imbalance this might produce. In some isolated cases, however, this has not happened and the result has been something akin to imprisonment. Conversely, maternity patients who are perhaps the least dependent on staff are one of the categories of patient who frequently criticise the care they receive.[27]

Another important factor in producing different responses is the age of the patient. Carstairs found that older people were more likely to express satisfaction with the hospital care they had received.[28] In the visiting survey at Hull we found too that the older the informant the more likely they were to say they were satisfied with the existing arrangements for visiting or indeed would prefer them to be reduced.[29] Clearly, experience of more restrictive regimes in the past has conditioned them to be more accepting now. I clearly remember one old lady whom I interviewed as part of the Manchester project, saying, in response to a question on the adequacy of visiting periods, that she appreciated anything the hospital permitted her; and what they permitted her was much more than she had been permitted in the past. A combination of elderly patients and great dependency may partially explain the rather sad picture of the geriatric hospitals found in the 1971 report of the Hospital Advisory Service.[30] There are no countervailing forces to push the point of equilibrium to a situation which is acceptable to those outside the immediate situation.

It follows from this that we can expect some younger patients to be less accepting of restrictions without an obvious medical rationale. In our study of patient reactions to hospital visiting times such a group was just discernible in our material.[31] One of the wards included in our sample was the male orthopaedic on which there was a number of young men who had had motorcycle accidents. They wanted to maintain their social contacts with other young people while in hospital. As far as visiting was concerned this attitude was clearly linked to a preference for more frequent visiting and fewer restrictions on the numbers allowed at any one time. Such patients as these could be said to have a very strict view of the authority conceded to the health service personnel, and consequently were more unwilling to accept restraints on freedom. This impressionistic evidence is supported by other studies. Carstairs found that the age group sixteen to forty-four were the least satisfied patients.[32]

Class is another variable which could be important in determining patient response to health care although Carstairs found there was no association between class and expressions of satisfaction with the service offered.[33] However, when asked to make critical comment, people from higher social groups were more likely to be forthcoming with one. This was particularly so with women. One word of explanation is required at this stage. In the Carstair's study critical comments were made, for example, about food. How does this kind of criticism fit into our hypothesis about a conflict of interest and objectives? It fits in this way. Food is given insufficient attention, according to the patients. It implies that their needs have not, in their view, been given sufficient weight. The staff, however, are not necessarily the beneficiaries – they, too, have to eat the food! On the other hand the trouble may be the insufficient attention given to its presentation on the ward. Complaints about food may fit our hypothesis in two ways. The conflicts of interest may not only be between staff and patients but between staff and those who provide the resources.

Food is not the only cause of complaint. Middle-class patients are probably more likely to challenge particular rules, for example, on the withholding of information.[34] It follows that a practice or a ward with a large middle-class component will probably have to have much more liberal rules on what information should be passed on to the patient. But this is not to say that where there are middle-class patients all rules will necessarily be challenged more often. On visiting arrangements, for example, a working-class patient, used to frequent contacts with the extended family, might prefer less restrictions on the number who can visit at any one time. A large gathering round the bed might be a more familiar and less daunting scene than the hospital preference for two at the bedside at one time: middle-class patients, less familiar with this type of social contact, might find these particular rules fall within their zone of acceptance.

Another important predictor of patient responses is the psychology of the patient. Regardless of class or age some patients seem to be happier when they are dependent. In a small study Coser has suggested that broadly speaking there were two patient orientations to hospital life.[35] First, there were those who enjoyed the care and attention they received. These patients were characterised by the ease with which they adapted to ward life, the emphasis they placed on the importance of the doctor's manner and a comparative lack of independence after discharge. The second group had an instrumental view of hospital regarding the clinical expertise as the most important component of their idea of a good doctor; were more likely to make suggestions for improvement of services when asked: and were more prepared to take up outside activities on discharge. Submissive patients who enjoy the primary care and attention may help to produce more restrictive regimes.

These then are some of the factors which would explain different responses of patients to health care. The objectives or needs (these words are almost interchangeable in this context) of different groups explain at least partially the different situations found in different parts of the health service. In some cases it may be explained by the countervailing pressure of the consumer, for example where they are articulate and informed. In most cases no doubt these needs are accommodated quite happily by the local managers.

CONCLUSION

The notion of equilibrium assumes a search for accommodation rather than conflict. We identified some of the factors that will determine the most appropriate point for the accommodation and that are likely to influence the future balance between interests of the various parties. At the moment the equilibrium is sometimes achieved by controllers of resources and staff in the service without too sound a knowledge of patient needs. A better appreciation of the patients' needs, differences between them and a recognition of the need for readjustments are the keys to successful management of staff/patient relationships in the future.

It is clear that consumers will accept rules which are not medically necessary as fair and reasonable. There have to be common meal times on wards to enable catering and nursing staff to operate effectively. Day patients, too, will have to accept that they may have to go rather later or earlier than they would wish because of the operational requirements of the ambulance service.

There will be conflicts of interest, of course. Staff have needs and objectives which they want met from employment. Older paediatric staff probably wanted children to be dependent on them. The parents' desire to be with their children, if realised, would lessen the chances of meeting this objective. In some cases staff training may take precedence over the need for a stable continuing relationship between doctor and patient as, for example, in mental subnormality.

There is perhaps another implication of this argument which deserves special mention. This is the need to particularise wherever possible. The evidence on the differences between patients strengthens the case for the delegation of authority downwards. For example, discretion to allow more than two visitors to the bedside of a working-class man used to constant interaction with his extended family is important in patient management. This assumes prior training of staff (or indoctrination!). Delegation of authority to staff who do not accept the rights of patients to have their interests considered (e.g. the psychiatric hospital scandals) would be disastrous.

19

Patient Management: Practical Issues

In this chapter we look at three issues in the field of patient management. The first two – the transition from person to patient and the care of the dying – are chosen to demonstrate the ways in which the equilibrium may have to be adjusted to accommodate patients' interests more effectively. We conclude by looking at the representation of patient interests in the new service.

I FROM PERSON TO PATIENT

The transition from person to patient is a traumatic one. In the case of admission into institutions it has been represented by Goffman and others as an attack on the patient's concept of himself.[1] One ceases to be a person and adopts the role of a patient. The transition is less obvious in the community health field, clinics or in out-patient departments. It is also less of a problem for patients who only stay in hospital for a short time. Yet even on these 'low profile' occasions the patient often feels stripped of his identity.

Certain features of the patient role may be dysfunctional even from a medical point of view. Institutional neurosis, with the difficulties this produces for discharge, is an obvious example. The inability of patients to absorb medical information about what to do after discharge may well be related to the dependent role in which they are often cast. Given, too, the pressure to reduce the length of stay in institutions more concurrence between patient and person roles may become increasingly necessary in the future.

Taylor has reported a pilot study on the impact of admission procedures on people becoming patients in seven psychiatric institutions in Britain.[2] The crucial moment in the process is the first contact with a member of staff. If the staff member has been notified of the arrival much is gained. If the staff member directs pleasantly and personally a jittery patient can be reassured.

Attention to detail of this type does not run counter to the staff interests.

The stark alternative to this situation is also described.[3] Confusion as to who the patient is and his purpose, and the damage of a greeting like ' "He's for Ward 4" implying parcel destination' with the implication that the patient cannot hear or if he can, he's a non-person anyway.[4] This approach may run counter to staff interests (or some of them). People are usually anxious when they seek medical advice and treatment, particularly if it involves admission to hospital. If poor reception arrangements make this anxiety worse then diagnosis and treatment may be made more difficult. The combination of anxiety and poor reception may explain why the patient can never remember those details which receptionists expect him to have at his fingertips. Human frailty may also explain why the exact date of previous visits, which of twenty different doctors one has seen, the date of X-rays and laboratory tests, index number, date of operation, who did it and name of next-of-kin are not always in the forefront of one's mind.

This is not just a matter of personalities and wise selection procedures. Different arrangements for reception may help. Taylor feels that ward responsibility for reception, investigation and assessment is more likely to produce acknowledgement of 'the newcomer's right to a personal life in the outside world'[5] because staff are constantly reminded of such an existence. If admission procedures are mainly the responsibility of the community services or other units in the hospital the interest of ward staff is narrowed to problems of socialisation. It may be that ward rather than specialist responsibility is inconvenient for staff, though it is unclear why this should be so. If it is, then a move to ward reception of patients would give less weight to the interests of staff and more to those of the patients.

At the moment centralised arrangements for reception find much favour. It is easy to see the advantages. Specialisation, use of clerical rather than scarce professional skills, and more effective collection of information are some of them.

It is also possible to see the dangers and the disadvantages to the patient who wants to be more of a person. Where there is a common reception point the receptionist will be anxious to obtain the fullest and most accurate documentation. He or she is judged on his or her success in obtaining it. The system encourages them to concentrate on procedure rather than helping people to adjust to being patients.

Ward or professional reception may be slightly better since it would be easier to build in other responsibilities and thus encourage a wider view of the patient's needs. The basis of specialisation will be different. It is with a group of people rather than one procedure affecting all patients. It accords too, with the view of Dr Howell who felt 'a consultant in geriatrics must take a wider view. He should regard the district as his battle ground'.[6] The reform of the health service will be an excellent opportunity to develop different bases of specialisation which encourage wider perspectives among staff.

It is worth recording that this is not a problem confined to Britain. Larkin and Phillips report an experiment in a hospital in the United States where a continuing care unit was established to help the reverse transition – from patient to person. There was, as in the U.K., a breakdown of care after discharge 'caused by a lack of sensitivity for the post-discharge needs of the patients and the absence of a co-ordinated effort on the part of staff to make timely and adequate preparation for continuity of care'.[7] Their solution was a unit whose staff were responsible for ensuring greater sensitivity to person rather than patient 'needs'.

Occasionally someone gives a glimpse of what it really feels like for some in the patient role. Williams has written very effectively of his experience as a polio patient in the 1950s. He refers to the habit of being addressed without a prefix '. . . one is reminded of the way in which prisoners are promptly denuded of their titles the moment they appear in the dock'.[8] Or the patients being treated as children by the nurse when 'one is scolded for not "eating up" one's dinner'.[9]

On the second occasion when he was in hospital it was primarily to receive physiotherapy. Since this was available only during the week he asked if he could go home at the weekends. The response was predictable and it proved impossible to arrange. 'This feeling of imprisonment in hospital is no doubt irrational and possibly childish . . . Hospitals could relieve these feelings . . . patients are not there to be given orders by them (doctors) or permissions; they are there to be given advice. They are not doctors' servants: the doctors are theirs, and should behave as such.'[10] This prescription must be the very antithesis of what many patients must feel during teaching rounds.

This very brief extract from Williams' account serves two purposes. First, it is a particular patient's perspective on what it really felt like to be on the receiving end of professional behaviour. Second, it suggests ways in which the patient's need for personalisation may be met without undermining the professional's need for defence mechanisms.

Administrative inconvenience or difficulties prevented his discharge for weekends. A greater willingness to accept inconvenience and difficulties on the part of staff may have meant more problems for them. It would have involved negotiations with the ambulance service which may have not taken kindly to the request. It may have generated considerable paper work when it seemed more profitable to use professional skills on professional duties. Yet, such a change would mean giving the patient's needs more consideration, without at the same time removing the defence mechanisms of detachment which is felt to be required for professional people. The five-day wards and out-patient surgery (which were not motivated by notions of patient convenience) are some of the developments which show how possible it was to meet Williams' request!

We accept that a problem for staff is the need to remain detached and not become personally involved in individual cases. The management problem is to strike the right balance between the professional need for detachment as a defence mechanism with a recognition of the individuality of the patient. It may be that the alternatives are not always mutually exclusive. We have referred above to Menzies' work. 'Sisters were deprived of the potential satisfaction in their roles' and many of them 'would like closer contact with the patients and more opportunity to use their nursing skills directly'. Administration and certain defence mechanisms against anxiety did not provide job satisfaction.[11]

The transition from person to patient is clearly a problem area. It can be made less of a problem by perhaps changing the basis of specialisation and responsibility for admission procedures. Such a change would bring in its wake probable disadvantages for staff.

Some may feel that this kind of change can only be wrought by groups representing patients' interests. Some may point to the community health councils and argue that this is what we can legitimately expect of them. We will look at this argument a little later. At this stage we can say that the past performance of representatives of the community as watchdogs of patient interests has not been particularly encouraging. We can expect more from an organisation of work which encourages staff to see that his ultimate objectives – good health – might be more easily realised by giving greater precedence to patients' interests in the institution itself. 'The present attitude towards patients encourages them to regress, minimises learning and perpetuates hospital reliance in Society.'[12]

II TERMINAL CARE

This soulless impersonal phrase is deliberately used to illustrate the point we have made above. It is a by-product of professional detachment. Anxiety is at its most acute where a patient is clearly dying. 'Terminal care' is a sufficiently impersonal phrase to provide some kind of defence against that anxiety.

Dying patients are, however, as much a part of successful patient management as the management of those who will recover from this particular episode. They will rapidly become a much more important part of patient management. Klein and Ashley have calculated, admittedly on the basis of some crude and arbitrary assumptions, that an extrapolation of current trends in the admission rates and length of stay of the elderly suggest that 'something like four-fifths of all hospital beds would be occupied by the elderly in 1992'.[13] No doubt the chronically sick and the old will form an even larger part of the caseload of the community health services too. 'Perhaps the time has come for the health services industry to balance its emphasis on life-saving services heavily orientated to short-term emergency care with the creation of a broad range of services geared towards helping people cope with the crises of transition, such as those produced by life-taking diseases'.[14] Such a shift would imply a higher priority to patients' needs, or at least the needs of this particular group.

This would involve care designed to emphasise the patient's identity. A label of 'incurable' can strip a person of his occupational and social status which are so important in his sense of identity. Anyone who returns to a place where they were formerly employed often find that they are only half-remembered and feel irrelevant to what is going on. They have become a non-person since they no longer have any relevance or status in the place. In miniature this must be what the dying patient must feel.

Practical expression can be given to a desire to sustain the individuality of the dying patient by organising work around what have been called the 'critical junctures' in the process of dying.[15] These junctures are:

1. Patient defined as dying.
2. Staff and patients make preparations for death.
3. The point at which there seems nothing more to do to prevent death.

4. The final descent ending in death.
5. The 'last hours'.
6. The death watch.
7. Death itself.

At all these stages the patient demands (or should do) considerable attention from staff. The timing of these 'junctures' can be planned, thus preventing, for example, the withdrawal of manpower from scheduled tasks with other patients. In terms of staff management, dying patterns should be determined by the staff of the unit and individuals trained to work to these specific patterns.[16]

This involves other changes on the part of staff. Avoidance techniques (e.g. conversational tactics which interrupt the patient), or management practices which incidentally make it difficult to raise matters with staff (e.g. job rotation) become suspect or require modification. It will not be easy. One only has to read the results of a small-scale survey by Strank to realise the stress of nursing the chronic sick and dying and the importance of avoiding too great an identification with individual patients. This was even more so where cytotoxic drugs were used with their disturbing side-effects.[17]

It is nevertheless another area of health care where the equilibrium between staff interests (protection from anxiety) and patient interests (a person rather than a patient) might be adjusted a little in favour of the latter. And given the attitudes to death in Britain today the pressure for change will have to come largely from staff. Public pressure, even through a community health council, is hardly likely on this point.

Another issue which raises the same sort of problems is the care of the unpopular patient. The professional ethics of the health service professions have until recently made it difficult for staff to admit such a problem exists. But the unpopular patient does exist and the possibility of rejection is now acknowledged by people in the service.[18]. A middle-class patient who has an instrumental attitude to health care demanding, for example, more information from doctors, is not infrequently classed as a 'trouble maker'. Or a dying patient who handles his or her illness in such a way that it provokes the maximum anxiety among staff, might be classified as 'selfish'. These, however, are normal defensive reactions which nevertheless make it more difficult for staff to 'personalise' their service.

It is possible to compensate for this phenomenon but with

possible disadvantages for the staff. It may, for example, involve changing tasks and disposition of personnel to allow staff who have not rejected the patient to form some kind of relationship with him. Cheadle reports that rejection is not total; the patient 'will always have a good proportion of staff to turn to . . .'[19] There are opportunities for staff to intervene *if* (a big *if*) they realise such an appreciation of the patient is developing. Ekdowi has reported that 'the opinion that a patient is difficult is slowly formed but once established and repeatedly expressed in nursing roles and medical records it rarely alters and may have a powerful influence on a patient's career in hospital'.[20] It is the slowness of the process which offers opportunities for intervention to head off or soften the judgement.

Some may feel the costs of changes of this type make such a shift not worthwhile. It would undermine the well-tried strategy of detachment and a more insecure staff may not be conducive to the efficient use of resources. It would also be difficult since the criterion of efficiency will push in the direction of greater routine and less attention to individual needs.

However, the decision to reform the National Health Service in 1974 was partly inspired by a desire to widen the appreciative settings of health personnel. The tripartite structure was seen to be responsible for the 'blinkers' which developed and the lack of attention to the total health needs of the patient. The change was presented as a beneficial one for patients though without affecting staff interests and objectives. The reform itself and in particular the introduction of the health service commissioner and the hospital advisory service carries with it the implication that greater efforts should be made to ensure more weight is given to patient interests.

This will involve training and education of staff to ensure that there is a move in this direction. Some may feel this is insufficient and that we need other ways to ensure the patients' case is heard at the crucial moments.

III PATIENTS' INTERESTS IN THE REFORMED HEALTH SERVICE

There are three 'official' institutions which might be said to represent the interests of patients in the new structure. First, there are the formal procedures for complaints including the health service commissioner and secondly, the community health councils. Since neither are in operation at the time of writing, comment on their effectiveness is necessarily speculative. The third one is the hospital advisory service (though it would be wrong to suggest that its sole purpose is to represent patients' interests).

In addition, a number of pressure groups representing patients have developed over the last five years. The Patients Association, and perhaps the more acceptable (officially) associations for mental health, welfare of children in hospital and age concern will have a considerable but unofficial influence on staff/patient relationships. Their impact is hardest to analyse since little is known of the relationship between their activities and decision-making in the service. It might not even be admitted that there is a relationship! We therefore concentrate on the official agencies for the representation of patient interests since most staff would admit to their existence and importance.

It may be thought that one other means of representing the consumer is conspicuous by its absence. Members of local health committees, regional hospital boards, hospital management committees and executive councils were supposed to safeguard and promote the interests of patients, as are their successors after 1974. We have excluded them from our list of institutions to safeguard patients' interests because of the limited impact of their predecessors! Perhaps Ely was an extreme case but the following quotation from the report on the hospital is a good illustration of their ineffectiveness in the role of patients' champion.

'Q. Have you been perfectly happy about what you have seen here?
A. Perfectly.
Q. In fact you did a long inspection of the hospital yesterday?
A. Yes.'[21]

The answers were given by a senior member of the management committee.

A similar situation existed at Whittingham. The minutes of a meeting at which student nurses complained about conditions at the hospital were suppressed before management committee members could see them. When they were brought to light two years later the committee 'reprimanded the chief male nurse and the matron; but the opportunity to deal with the problems raised was missed'.[22]

Members in both cases were quite unable to protect patients' interests even when the pendulum had clearly swung too far in favour of staff convenience. This is not a view confined to those who look at the service from the outside. 'After seven years as a member of a regional hospital board I am convinced that we would have a far better health service today if the consumer had had an effective voice . . .'[23] Unfortunately there is no obvious reason why members will be more effective than their predecessors in the hospital service were.

The most interesting and possibly the most influential of the three official ways of representing the patients' interests is the hospital advisory service. Since it was established in November, 1969, its work so far seems to have had a fair reception. Its composition of practising health service staff gives it a strong claim for a good hearing from personnel in the service. Its reports are not uncritical (thus avoiding the charge of white-washing) and are constructive. The confidentiality, though broken in some instances by some newspapers, should breed confidence in staff who wish to be frank in discussion. For the top management of the service the reports provide an effective early-warning system. One hopes that the detachment from a particular situation which is being inspected produces a lower level of identification with staff interests, and a correspondingly higher one with those of patients where this is appropriate.

Formal complaints machinery is another medium to ensure patients are correctly treated. This did exist in the unreformed health service. In the executive council sector, for example, patients could complain to a service committee of seven members.[24] Of these, three were representative of the profession, three laymen of the executive council with a mutually acceptable chairman. Complaints were few. Successful complaints were even fewer. It is hard to believe that, for example, the vast number of patient–general practitioner contacts in a year produce so little criticism. Formal procedures are unlikely to encourage complaints of a transient, minor but irritating nature. And it is at this minor level that patients' interests (e.g. about the length of time one spends in GP's waiting rooms) could perhaps be given more weight and for which formal procedures seem inappropriate.

A similar objection applies to the health service commissioner. He is going to be a court of appeal. Only when patients, or relatives or staff acting on their behalf, have exhausted the other formal machinery, and are not satisfied with the replies they have received will they have a right of access to the commissioner. The commissioner's remit for those cases which reach him will be those cases where an individual 'has suffered injustice or hardship through maladministration, or through a failure to provide necessary treatment or care . . .'[25] Certainly there will be a countervailing force where there was none before. Yet he is unlikely to influence the rather intangible areas which the patient may think important – human relations, less regimentation. The better accommodation of patients' interests at this level will owe very little to these formal channels of complaint. We have mentioned already the reluctance of patients to complain. Formal complaints procedures are hardly likely to encourage them. Perhaps the commissioner's greatest value will be the knowledge of his existence which may prevent the service becoming too orientated to staff interests.

What of the new community health councils? To the extent they are modelled on the consumer councils in the nationalised industry they are unlikely to be an effective watchdog. It is hard to see them, for example, having much influence on the choice between centralisation of scarce and expensive medical resources and inconvenience to the public, particularly in rural areas. Or again on those management decisions where there is a clear conflict between efficient use of resources and the patient's notions of comfort. As an illustration of this second dilemma we turn again to the introduction of the forty-eight hour maternity discharge scheme in Bradford. The change provided the margin of resources necessary for other developments. Cohen looked at the same experiment from the perspective of the mother. 'Both obstetric and public health personnel express high satisfaction with this method of delivering three times the number of babies in the same old buildings – and none the worse for it . . .' A young teacher thought back, '. . . it was such a rush, the whole business, everyone pushing and chivvying me to get on with the job; and when he was born, the milk wouldn't come but they just said: "Oh well, the District Nurse'll put you right"; and she had 'flu, so by the time another one got here he was on Cow and Gate.'[26] It is at this level that the conflict between the interests of efficiency and the patients is most real. It may be that most mothers prefer to be at home after two days in hospital. This is not the point. A change on this scale is more likely to come from an obstetrician who wants to use his beds more intensively than a patient pressure group.

Our concern here is the proper balance between the interests of efficiency, represented by managers, and those of the individual patient. There is a real danger that the interests of the patient will be given too little weight because of the absence of adequate representation. If so, it is hard to see the community health council as presently envisaged being able to do much about it. Kirk has argued that their position may be strengthened by a different method of appointment and a link with the health service commissioner, who would in turn be given wider terms of reference.[27] He feels that instead of being partially appointed by the area health authorities members should be appointed by a national body to emphasise their independence. Appointment by a body with management responsibility for the service will cast doubt on this and may inhibit members. The link with the commissioners would, too, emphasise independence and clarify their role as patients or the public's champions.[28]

Even if these changes were agreed it is probable, at least in certain areas, that the community health councils will be weak. To view them as adequate representation for patients' interests either at a strategic planning or operational level would be unwise. Staff themselves will still have to act as watchdogs against too great a precedence being given to their own interests. It will often be their job to initiate change to achieve a better deal for patients. It is hard to see, for example, a community health council having as much impact on the treatment of maternity patients[29] and the organisation of the timing of routine on wards or the visiting and care of children in hospitals as did the committees largely composed of professionals.[30] In another problem area – waiting in out-patient departments – it is again hard to see a community health member winning a discussion with a consultant who overbooks or an out-patient sister who operates a tacit 'first come, first served' system. An active manager who feels patients should not be kept waiting so long will do better. Community health councils, even if they are more effective than we suppose, do not absolve staff from their responsibilities.

If the major responsibility, in spite of the creation of these new bodies, for a fair balance between staff and patient interests remains with staff they may rightly ask what it is that patients really want (although more often they insist they already know). Without this information it is difficult to strike an acceptable or fair balance where interests conflict. In these situations there is a real danger that the articulate may be unwisely taken as representative of a wider body of opinion (as they are in many walks of life). Even if the articulate are representative of the silent majority, a minority of patients may feel their vital interests ignored.

The difficulty of divining public reaction does not mean attempts should not be made to assess it. It underlines an earlier point we made. Response to patient needs has to be more sophisticated and flexible if a satisfactory balance between the interests of the different participants is to be achieved. There have to be different balances and arrangements in different places. The prime responsibility for a successful *modus vivendi* will be that of managers in the service who as before will have to compensate for the weakness of institutions that are supposed to promote and safeguard patients' interests. No doubt in most cases they will continue to perform this function more than adequately.

20

Management in the Integrated Health Service

Administrative reform is not a panacea for the problems which beset those who in any sense manage the health service. There will not be a large increase in the resources made available and problems of co-ordination will not suddenly disappear. Indeed for a considerable period of time things may get worse before they get better. This will not only be due to the confusion which surrounds any organisational reform. New colleagues who will be feeling each other out and are uncertain of their position in the new structure may often be less forthcoming than they were when employed by different authorities.

One of the greatest dangers to the success of the new service is the reaction when it is finally realised that some of the more unrealistic expectations are unlikely to be realised. The delay in the full implementation of the new management structure will make this reaction probable sooner rather than later. Managers must be on their guard against these unrealistic expectations and over-reactions when they are not realised and be clear about the ways in which reorganisation is likely to help.

The new management structure will not solve problems by itself. It offers a more helpful framework in which to tackle those management problems which have always existed. Hopefully the abolition of formal boundaries between community and hospital services will permit enterprising managers to deploy their resources, particularly staff, more flexibly and effectively; the provision of a common reference point at local level will encourage quicker decisions on issues affecting both sectors; and planning the development of both services will provide a better balance between the two. The success of the reform depends on how these opportunities are taken.

More will be expected of managers in the service. We have discussed at some length the pressures on them to improve efficiency. The improvements in the quality of management

189

information, particularly in the field of norms of good practice, provide increasingly effective measures not only of the effectiveness of the service but the efficiency with which resources are used. They provide a useful starting point from which to monitor the performance of managers.

It will be legitimate to expect managers to anticipate future problem areas and take action accordingly. We have suggested that patient–staff relationships will fall into this category. The increasing proportion of elderly and chronic sick in case-loads will require everyone to be on his or her guard against situations where patients' interests are given too little consideration and to respond differently to the management of death. We can expect too that younger age groups may not so willingly accept arrangements which their elders took for granted and regarded as immutable.

It adds up to a very challenging environment in which to work. For some it may be a very threatening one. It is possible that the working environment may be made even more challenging by some features of the new management structure which might place bigger obstacles in the path of the manager.

One of the causes of poor co-ordination is the manoeuvring for power and status by the occupational groups in the service. The growing barriers between, for example, the nursing and medical professions are now a matter of official concern[1] (though the explanations of this are different to the ones we have offered). The development of parallel hierarchies for various groups – a trend underlined by the proposed management structure for the new service – may make it harder for managers to overcome these barriers. They may make for improvements within occupational groups, for example between community and hospital nurses. However, without more mechanisms for cross-over points below district level these improvements may be at the expense of lateral contacts within the organisation. If this is so then it will not only produce or perhaps intensify problems of day-to-day co-ordination of services, but the sense of identification with the organisation as a whole may well be impaired. Without that sense of identification decisions about budgets, allocations of the increment and savings between departments, may be based less often on the criterion of efficiency and more often on notions of adequacy. The pathologist who wants money for a development in his department must see that it can only be provided at the expense, say, of something in the community nursing field. He must be exposed to the claims of others in addition to his colleagues in the Cogwheel structure.

Hopefully the health care planning teams may provide this wider perspective for some.

Among the many whom we have identified as having some managerial responsibilities there may still be questions about the expertise and training required to cope with such a challenging environment. Apprehensions may be increased by the conspicuous absence in this book of simple answers to common management problems. Most of us (including those who refuse to supply them) yearn for universally applicable, simple, straightforward answers to complex problems.

Recognition that there are no panaceas, that new techniques need careful evaluation before being employed, and that experience in handling people is still important means that the managers do not meet these challenges unaided. If they can add to these essentials a broader appreciation of people in organisations and a greater commitment to efficiency at the expense of adequacy, then will they be able to take full advantage of the opportunities offered by the integration of the health services.

Notes

CHAPTER 1

1 Department of Health and Social Security, *National Health Service reorganisation*, Consultative document (1971), pp. 1–2.
2 Department of Health and Social Security, *Management arrangements for the reorganised National Health Service* (HMSO, 1972).
3 For example:
    (i) Ministry of Health, Scottish Home and Health Department, *Report of the committee on senior nursing staff structure* (Salmon Report), (HMSO, 1966).
    (ii) Department of Health and Social Security; Scottish Home and Health Department; Welsh Office, *Report of the working party on management structure in the local authority nursing services* (1969).
    (iii) Department of Health and Social Security, *First and second reports of the joint working party on the organisation of medical work in hospitals* (HMSO, 1967 and 1972).
    (iv) G. P. E. Howard (Chairman), *The shape of hospital management in 1980* (King Edward's Hospital Fund for London, 1967).
4 The consultative document, op. cit., p. 2.
5 D. Williams, 'The administrative contribution of the nursing sister', *Public Administration*, Vol. 47, p. 307.
6 There is a considerable literature on this subject. For a balanced view see T. Lupton, *Management and the social sciences* (an Administrative Staff College publication, 1966), and M. Kogan, 'Management efficiency and the social services: a review article', *British Journal of Social Work*, Vol. 1, No. 1, pp. 105–21.
7 A. A. MacIver in *Modern hospital management*, J. F. Milne and N. W. Chaplin (eds.), (The Institute of hospital administrators, 1969).
8 E. Jaques, 'Organisational structure and role relationships', *Nursing Times*, Vol. 67, No. 5, pp. 154–7.
9 Ibid.
10 Members of some departments would have greater personal autonomy and be less subject to bureaucratic style of supervision, and heads of departments would therefore be less directly responsible for their work.
11 D. V. Donnison, V. Chapman *et al.*, *Social policy and administration* (Allen & Unwin, 1965), p. 234.

CHAPTER 2

1 Enoch Powell, *A new look at medicine and politics* (Pitman Medical, 1966), p. 20.
2 H. Miller, 'Is there an alternative?', BBC third programme (1 December 1966).
3 H. Travis, *20th Anniversary Conference of the National Health Service, Report* (HMSO, 1968), p. 32.

4 Spectator, 'Money and management', *The Hospital*, Vol. 64, No. 8, p. 380.
5 B.M.A. Planning Unit, 'Priorities in medicine', *British Medical Journal*, Vol. 1, No. 5636 (1969), p. 107.
6 *The Hospital*, Vol. 66, No. 12, p. 406.
7 *Lancet*, Vol. 1 for 1970, p. 25.
8 Royal Commission on Medical Education, *Report*, 1965–8 (Todd Report), Cmnd. 3569 (HMSO, 1968).
9 Arthur Seldon, 'Crisis in the Welfare State', *Encounter* (December 1967).
10 D. Mechanic, *Medical sociology* (The Free Press, 1968), p. 337.
11 R. Crossman, Public Lecture at the University of Hull, 22 January 1971.
12 Enoch Powell, op. cit., pp. 17–18.
13 *The Hospital and Health Service Review*, Vol. 68, No. 1, 'Health service expenditure.' Quoting Office of Health Economics, p. 25.
14 *Public Expenditure to 1975/6*, Cmnd. 4829 (HMSO, 1971), Table 1.2.
15 W. Godley and C. Taylor, 'The Public sectors' rising claim on resources', *The Times* (17 February 1971).
16 B. Abel Smith, *An international study of health expenditure*, Public Health Papers 32 (World Health Organisation, Geneva, 1967).

CHAPTER 3

1 *The Hospital and Health Service Review*, Vol. 68, No. 1, 'Health service expenditure'. Quoting *Office of Health Economics*, p. 25.
2 Ibid.
3 Ministry of Health and Department of Health and Social Security, annual reports.
4 *Public expenditure to 1975/6*, Cmnd. 4829 (HMSO, 1971), p. 52.
5 D. A. T. Griffiths, 'Inequalities and management in the N.H.S.', *The Hospital*, Vol. 67, No. 7, pp. 229/30.
6 Ibid., p. 231.
7 N. Bosanquet, 'Inequalities in the health service', *New Society*, No. 450.
8 R. Titmuss and B. Abel Smith, *The cost of the National Health Service in England and Wales* (Cambridge University Press, 1956).
9 R. Klein and J. Ashley, 'Old age health', *New Society*, No. 484.
10 *Public Expenditure to 1975/6*, op. cit., p. 52.
11 W. W. Holland, 'Clinicians and the use of medical resources', *The Hospital*, Vol. 67, No. 7, p. 236.
12 We are not suggesting that this did not happen in this case. We are talking hypothetically about the reactions of management to this type of increased demand.
13 R. Crossman, Public Lecture at the University of Hull, 22 January 1971.

CHAPTER 4

1 Hansard, *Parliamentary Debates. Commons*, Vol. 740, column 1559.
2 B.M.A. planning unit, 'Priorities in medicine', *British Medical Journal*, Vol. 1, No. 5636 (1969), p. 106.
3 Enoch Powell, *A new look at medicine and politics* (Pitman Medical, 1966), p. 20.
4 *Nursing Mirror* (27 October 1967), p. 88.

5 'News of the week', *Nursing Times*, Vol. 65, No. 52, p. 636.
6 Leader article: 'Is there a shortage of nurses?', *Nursing Times*, Vol. 67, No. 41, p. 1263.
7 Report of the Committee on Nursing, Cmnd. 5115 (HMSO, 1972), para. 5.
8 Ibid., para. 447.
9 Ibid., para. 448.
10 T. G. Booth and M. A. Steane, 'Hospital practice: a comparison of staffing difficulties in several professions', *Occupational Therapy*, Vol. 33, No. 12, pp. 9–14.
11 Report of the Committee on Nursing, op. cit., para. 447.
12 D. A. T. Griffiths, 'Inequalities and management in the N.H.S.', *The Hospital*, Vol. 67, No. 7, p. 231.
13 N. Bosanquet, 'Inequalities in the health service', *New Society*, No. 450, p. 810. This view conflicts with the conclusion of the Briggs Committee as far as nursing staff were concerned, p. 447.
14 Annual Report of the Department of Health and Social Security, 1969 (HMSO, 1970), p. 33.
15 A. D. Bonham Carter, 20th Anniversary of N.H.S., *Report* (HMSO, 1968), p. 66.
16 Annual report of the General Nursing Council, 1966–7, p. 14.

CHAPTER 5

1 D. Paige and K. Jones, *Health and welfare services in Britain in 1975* (Cambridge University Press, 1966), p. 106.
2 R. F. L. Logan (1963), *Proceedings of the Royal Society of Medicine*, 56, 309.
3 G. Forsyth, *Doctors and state medicine. A study of the British health service* (Pitman Medical, London, 1966), p. 69.
4 J. O. Miller, B. Fevber, 'Health manpower in the 1960's, *Hospitals* (Journal of the American Hospital Association), Vol. 45, p. 69.
5 *The Hospital*, Vol. 66, No. 7, p. 221. An editorial comment with references to a talk by Sir Bruce Fraser at the Hospital Centre.
6 20th Anniversary of the N.H.S., *Report* (HMSO, 1968), p. 71.
7 J. M. Last, 'Community demand for doctors in the next ten years', *British Medical Journal* (1969), No. 5646, p. 769/72.
8 The evidence for this assertion is discussed more fully in Chapter 18.
9 An interview with T. Stewart Hamilton, *Hospitals*, Vol. 43, p. 54.

CHAPTER 6

1 Enoch Powell, *A new look at medicine and politics* (Pitman Medical, 1966), pp. 19–20.
2 H. Simon, *Administrative behavior* (The Free Press, paperback edition, 1965), pp. 212–13.
3 Enoch Powell, op. cit., pp. 15–16.
4 Enoch Powell, op. cit., p. 16.
5 J. Butterworth, *Hospital efficiency*, 'Productivity now' (Pergamon Press, 1969), pp. 55–70.
6 R. G. Walker, W. R. Miller and I. G. McClean, *A study of the work of*

hospital junior medical staff, Scottish Health Service Studies, No. 10 (Scottish Home and Health Department, 1969).

7 M. S. Feldstein, *Economic analysis for health service efficiency* (North Holland Publishing Company, Amsterdam, 1967), Chapter 2.

8 D. Adlington, 'Hospital efficiency and morale', *British Hospital Journal and Social Service Review*, Vol. 79, No. 4137, pp. 1446–7.

CHAPTER 7

1 M. Skeet, *A digest of Home from hospital* (The Dan Mason Research Committee, 1970), p. 8.

2 S. Levine and P. White, 'Exchange as a conceptual framework for a study of interorganisational relationships', *Administrative Science Quarterly* (March 1961), pp. 583–601.

3 J. J. Jarvis *et al.*, 'Towards an integrated service: a description of the integration of the maternity service in the Doncaster County Borough', *The Hospital*, Vol. 67, No. 2, pp. 49–51.

4 C. V. Ruckley *et al.*, 'Team approach to early discharge and outpatient surgery', *Lancet*, Vol. 1 for 1971, pp. 177–80.

CHAPTER 8

1 Department of Health and Social Security, Consultative document, *National Health Service reorganisation* (1971), p. 2.

2 E. Jaques, 'Producing the managers', *The Hospital*, Vol. 65, No. 7, p. 241.

3 S. G. Hill, in *Modern hospital management*, J. F. Milne and N. W. Chaplin (eds.), (The Institute of Hospital Administrators, 1969), p. 67.

4 A. A. MacIver, in *Modern hospital management*, ibid., p. 520.

5 A. A. MacIver, ibid., p. 526.

6 J. A. Spencer, *Management in hospitals* (Faber 1967), p. 39.

7 G. F. L. Packwood, 'The hospital secretary role', *The Hospital and Health Services Review*, Vol. 68, No. 3, pp. 85–8.

8 E. Jaques, 'Organisational structure and role relationships', *Nursing Times*, Vol. 67, No. 5, p. 155.

9 D. Silverman, *The theory of organisations* (Heinemann, 1970), p. 141.

10 T. Burns and G. M. Stalker, *The management of innovation* (Tavistock, 1966), p. 6.

11 By, for example, G. L. Ellis and D. M. Williams, 'Status in hospitals', *British Hospital Journal and Social Service Review*, Vol. 77, No. 4040, pp. 1792–3.

12 M. Steane and J. G. Booth, *Pharmaceutical Journal*, Vol. 202, No. 549, pp. 83–6.

13 D. Silverman, op. cit., p. 208.

14 J. A. Spencer, op. cit., p. 38.

15 Ibid., p. 38.

16 T. Burns and G. M. Stalker, op. cit., *passim*.

17 Ibid., p. 5.

18 Ibid., p. 6.

19 J. A. Spencer, op. cit., p. 39.

20 D. Williams, 'Diagnosing management training needs', *The Hospital*, Vol. 63, No. 3, pp. 100–2.

196 *Managing the Health Service*

21 *B.M.J.* Leading article, 'Practicalities of nursing', Vol. 3, No. 5774 (4 July 1971).
22 I. E. P. Menzies, 'A case study in the functioning of social systems as a defence against anxiety', *Human Relations*, Vol. 13, No. 2. pp. 95–121.
23 Ibid.

CHAPTER 9

1 Enoch Powell, *A new look at medicine and politics* (Pitman Medical, 1966), pp. 17–19.
2 C. Montacute in *Modern hospital management*, J. F. Milne and N. W. Chaplin (eds.) (The Institute of hospital administrators, 1969), p. 361.
3 After 1 April 1974 unspent balances will be transferable to the next financial year. White paper, *National Health Service reorganisation*, Cmnd. 5055 (HMSO, 1972), para. 158.
4 Report of discussion at an IHA conference, *The Hospital*, Vol. 65, No. 7, p. 240.
5 Management services (*NHS*), *Guide to good practice in hospital administration* (HMSO, 1970), p. 61.

CHAPTER 10

1 A warning also sounded by G. McLachlan (ed.) in *Challenges for change* (O.U.P. for Nuffield Provincial Hospitals Trust, 1971).
2 A. K. Rice, *The Enterprise and its environment* (Tavistock, 1971), p. 257.
3 I. Harper and R. L. Simpson, 'Women and bureaucracy in the semi-professions' in *The semi-professions and their organisation.* (The Free Press, 1969), pp. 199–200.
4 D. Donnison and V. Chapman *et al.*, *Social Policy and Administration* (Allen & Unwin, 1965), p. 234.
5 J. A. Spencer, *Management in hospitals* (Faber, 1967), p. 39.
6 Ibid., p. 38.
7 See chapter 8, p. 63–4.
8 G. L. Cohen, *What's wrong with hospitals?* (A Penguin special, 1964), p. 70.
9 Department of Health and Social Security, *Children in hospital: maintenance of family links and prevention of abandonment*, circular number HM(72), 2.
10 Secretary of State for Social Services, *Report of the Farleigh Hospital Committee of Inquiry*, Cmnd. 4557 (HMSO, 1971), para. 120.
11 Sir George Godber, 'Hospital and community: The pattern of medical care' Paper given to the third regional conference of the International Hospital Federation, September/October 1970.
12 L. Landon *et al.*, *Lancet*, Vol. 11 for 1971, No. 7722, pp. 480–2. The description that follows is based on this article.
13 Ibid. The cost was 70p per test in May 1971.
14 M. E. Gifford, 'A do-it-yourself CDH pram', *Nursing Times*, Vol. 67, No. 26, p. 806.
15 Dr A. Baker, *Report of the Hospital Advisory Service.* (HMSO, 1971), para. 60.
16 A. L. Amsden, 'Anatomy of achievement. What the nurses did.' *Nursing Times*, Vol. 67, No. 22, pp. 672–3.

17 J. Davies, *An evaluation of first-line management courses for ward sisters in the Manchester region: a study of management in its organisational context* (Centre for Business Research, Manchester, 1971).

CHAPTER 11

1 D. Mechanic, *Medical sociology* (The Free Press, 1968), p. 419.
2 Sir G. Godber, 'Hospital and Community. The pattern of medical care'. Paper given to the third regional conference of the International Hospital Federation. September/October 1970.
3 A. Etzioni, *The semi-professions and their organisation* (The Free Press, 1969).
4 A phrase borrowed from A. Etzioni. 'A basis for comparative analysis of complex organisations.' In *A sociological reader on complex organisations* (Holt, Rinehart & Winston, 1970), pp. 71–5.
5 H. J. Dellar and S. C. Haywood, unpublished research.
6 D. Mechanic, op. cit., p. 422.
7 *Report of the Farleigh Hospital Committee of Inquiry*, Cmnd. 4557 (HMSO, 1971), para. 79.
8 D. Donnison *et al.*, *Social Policy and Administration* (Allen & Unwin, 1965), p. 238.
9 Ibid., p. 239.
10 This is a speculative analysis and in no way purports to be a description of what actually happened.
11 Which did not happen. The illustration is being used as a basis for discussion on possible courses of action. The general discussion does not purport to be a description of events or a criticism of the officers involved.
12 The first report on the Hospital Advisory Service indicated this was a fairly common problem. Dr A. Baker, *Report of the Hospital Advisory Service* (HMSO, 1971), para. 83.

CHAPTER 12

1 R. Elkin and D. L. Cornick in *Social work administration*, H. A. Schatz (ed.) (Council on Social Work Education, New York, 1970), p. 366.
2 H. Simon, *Administrative Behavior* (The Free Press, paperback edition, 1965), p. 39.
3 J. A. Spencer, *Management in Hospitals* (Faber, 1967), p. 109.
4 H. Simon, op. cit., pp. 212–14.

CHAPTER 13

1 This section again concentrates on the type of management information made available to the pre-reform hospital service. The reason behind this is the organisational model adopted for the integrated health service. Life after 1974 will be much more similar to that which existed in the hospital service before reform, than to that in the other two arms of the tripartite service.
2 Hospital Administrative Staff College, King Edward's Hospital Fund for London, *Management Audit* (1966).

198   *Managing the Health Service*

3 M. S. Feldstein, *Economic analysis for health service efficiency* (North-Holland Publishing Company, Amsterdam, 1967), Chapter 2.
4 Ibid., Chapter 2.
5 Ministry of Health, *Annual Report for 1967*, Cmnd. 3702 (HMSO 1968), p. 49.
6 C. Montacute, *Costing and efficiency in hospitals*. (O.U.P., for Nuffield Provincial Hospitals Trust, 1969), p. 114.
7 Ibid., Table 17.
8 Ibid., p. 114.
9 Management Services (NHS), *Guide to good practices in hospital administration*, Department of Health and Social Security (HMSO, 1970).
10 Ibid., p. 66.
11 Ibid., p. 89.
12 Ibid., p. 29.
13 Ibid., p. 61.
14 Ibid., p. 6.
15 Department of Health and Social Security circular 13/72.
16 R. Stewart and J. Sleeman. Continuously under review. Occasional papers on social administration. No. 20 (G. Bell & Sons, 1967), p. 59.
17 'Efficient management', *The Hospital*, Vol. 63, No. 7, p. 251.
18 'Management audit', *The Hospital and Health Services Review*, Vol. 68, No. 1, p. 24.
19 H. Simon, *Administrative Behavior* (The Free Press, 1965), p. xxiv.
20 Ibid., p. xxiv.
21 M. W. Cuming, 'Management by objectives', *The Hospital*, Vol. 64, No. 4, pp. 122–4.
22 Ibid., p. 122.
23 Which may or may not have been so in this case.
24 W. W. Holland, *The Hospital*, Vol. 67, No. 7, pp. 236–9.
25 Management Services (NHS), op. cit., para. 27.
26 J. Pantall and J. Elliot, 'Can research aid hospital management?', *The Hospital*, Vol. 63, No. 10, p. 384.
27 H. Simon, op. cit., p. 215.
28 Sir Arnold France, then permanent Secretary to the Ministry of Health. Report of an address to the National Association of Group Secretaries, 1966, *The Hospital*, Vol. 62, No. 7, p. 346.

CHAPTER 14

1 J. Pantall and J. Elliot, 'Can research aid hospital management?', *The Hospital*, Vol. 63, No. 9, p. 337.
2 B. Moores, 'In Search of motivation', *The Hospital*, Vol. 67, No. 3, pp. 75–80.
3 Management services (NHS), *Guide to good practices in hospital administration*, DHSS (HMSO, 1970), p. 27.
4 'Community demand for doctors in the next ten years', *B.M.J.*, Vol. 1, 1969, No. 5646, p. 771.
5 Dr J. O. F. Davies, 20th Anniversary Conference of the N.H.S., *Report* (HMSO, 1968), p. 62.
6 Management services (N.H.S.), op. cit., p. 17.
7 Ibid., p. 29.

8 Ibid., p. 17.
9 No easy money for the NHS, *Hospital Management*, Vol. 33, No. 401, p. 290.

CHAPTER 15

1 E. Jaques, Organisational structure and role relationships, *Nursing Times*, Vol. 67, No. 5, pp. 154–5.
2 A. M. Bowey, Organisational theory and hospital administration, *The Hospital*, Vol. 67, No. 11, p. 380.
3 D. McGregor, 'Changing patterns in human relations', *Conference Board Management Record*, Vol. 12, No. 9, p. 366 (quoted by R. Stewart in *The reality of management* (Pan Books, 1967), p. 114).
4 H. Simon, *Administrative behavior* (The Free Press, 1965), p. 111.
5 J. K. Galbraith, *The new industrial state* (Hamish Hamilton, 1967), p. 130.
6 H. Simon, op. cit., p. 115.
7 Ibid., p. 205.
8 J. K. Galbraith, op. cit., p. 131.
9 Ibid., p. 132.
10 Ibid., p. 132.

CHAPTER 16

1 R. Stewart, *The Reality of management* (Pan Books 1967), p. 113, quoting Robert L. Kahn, 'Human relations on the shop floor' in *Human relations and modern management*, E. M. Hugh Jones (ed.), pp. 49–51 (North Holland Publishing Company, Amsterdam, 1958).
2 M. Schofield, 'The unwanted child', *The Hospital*, Vol. 67, No. 3, p. 81.
3 R. Stewart, op. cit., p. 115.
4 H. Brinton, 'Cut price health', *The Lancet*, Vol. 11 for 1971, No. 7726, pp. 499–700.
5 M. Schofield, op. cit., p. 81.

CHAPTER 17

1 T. Lupton, *Management and the social sciences* (Hutchinson, 1966) (An Administrative Staff College publication), p. 74.
2 P. M. Blau and W. R. Scott. *Formal organisations* (Routledge and Kegan Paul) pp. 64–74.
3 P. M. Blau, and W. R. Scott, op. cit., p. 69, Quoting work by W. Q. Benis *et al.*, *Administration Science Quarterly*, 2 (1958), pp. 481–500.
4 S. C. Haywood and H. J. Dellar. 'The nursing view of management', *British Hospital Journal and Social Service Review*, Vol. LXXXI, No. 4215, pp. 223–4.
5 S. C. Haywood and H. J. Dellar, unpublished paper. 'Part-time nurses'.
6 Ibid.
7 P. M. Blau and W. R. Scott, op. cit., pp. 69–70. 'Her performance is observable only to her colleagues in the immediate work group . . . The nurse who is committed to her professional skills expresses a high loyalty to her work group since only this group can give this praise and recognition for work well done.'

8 R. W. Revans, *Standards for morale: cause and effect in hospitals* (O.U.P. for Nuffield Provincial Hospitals Trust, 1964).

9 Department of Health and Social Security, Welsh Office, *Progress on Salmon* (1972).

10 T. M. Higham, 'Basic psychological factors in communication', *Occupational Psychology*, Vol. 31 (January 1957), pp. 4–5. Quoted by Charles Redfield, 'The theory of communication', *Social Work Administration* (Council on Social Work Education, N.Y., 1970), p. 179.

11 Ibid., pp. 178–9.

12 Ibid., p. 178.

13 P. M. Blau and W. R. Scott, op. cit., p. 128.

14 J. F. Milne and N. W. Chaplin (eds.), *Modern Hospital Management* (The Institute of hospital administrators, 1969), p. 75.

15 P. M. Blau and W. R. Scott, op cit., p. 131.

16 H. E. Leigh, G. F. Wieland, J. A. Anderson, 'The hospital internal communication project', *Lancet*, Vol. 1. for 1971, pp. 1005–9. Also *Changing hospitals: a report on the Hospital Internal Communications Project*, G. F. Weiland and H. Leigh (eds.), assisted by E. Barnes (Tavistock, 1971).

17 H. E. Leigh *et al.*, op. cit., p. 1005.

18 Ibid., p. 1007.

19 Ibid., p. 1005.

20 Charles Redfield, op. cit., p. 179.

21 Ibid., p. 179.

22 T. Lupton, op. cit., p. 69.

23 J. Pantall and J. Elliot, 'Can research aid hospital management?' A series of articles in *The Hospital* (June/July/August 1965 and September, October, December 1967). This quotation is from Vol. 63, No. 9, pp. 336–7.

24 A. W. Miles and D. Smith, *Joint consultation; defeat or opportunity* (King Edward's Hospital Fund for London, 1968).

25 J. M. Thompson, 'Survival of joint consultation', *British Hospital Journal and Social Service Review*, Vol. 79, No. 4138, p. 1498.

26 T. Lupton, op. cit., p. 69.

27 J. Pantal *et al.*, op. cit.

28 Ibid., p. 335.

29 J. Pantal *et al.*, *The Hospital*, Vol. 63, No. 12, p. 464.

30 J. D. Harvey, 'Toward more effective utilisation of manpower', *Hospitals*, Vol. 43, 1 January 1969.

31 F. Herzberg, *Work and the nature of man* (World Publishing Company, 1966).

32 L. Trotter and G. B. Adshead, 'A practical experiment in hospital personnel management', *The Hospital*, Vol. 64, No. 12, pp. 424–8.

33 Ibid., p. 425.

34 Ibid., p. 427.

35 Ibid., p. 427.

36 See for example M. W. Cuming, 'Labour-Turnover', *The Hospital*, Vol. 66, No. 11, p. 381.

37 L. Trotter and G. B. Adshead, op. cit., p. 424.

38 There are many books which present this case. Some of the more helpful ones are: O. McGregor, *The human side of the enterprise* (McGraw-Hill, 1960); R. Likert, *New patterns of management* (McGraw-Hill, 1961); J. A. C. Brown, *The social psychology of industry* (Penguin, 1964).

39 P. M. Blau and W. R. Scott, op. cit., p. 148.
40 Ibid., p. 142.
41 Ibid., pp. 144–5.
42 P. M. Blau and W. R. Scott, op. cit., pp. 163–4.
43 Ibid., p. 149.
44 Ibid., p. 151–3.
45 L. Trotter and G. B. Adshead, op. cit., p. 424.
46 See for example R. Blauner, 'Work satisfaction and industrial trends'. In A. Etzioni, *Sociological reader on complex organisations* (Holt, Rinehart, 1970), pp. 223–49.
47 T. Lupton, op. cit., p. 73.
48 Ibid., pp. 157–9.
49 Ibid., pp. 153–7.
50 P. M. Blau and W. R. Scott, op. cit., p. 154.
51 B. S. Georgepoulus and F. C. Mann, *The community general hospital* (Macmillan, 1962).
52 T. Tannenbaum and W. Schmidt, 'How to choose a leadership pattern', *Harvard Business Review*, Vol. 36, No. 2, pp. 95–101.
53 H. D. Stein in *Social work administration*, op. cit. 'Administrative leadership in complex service organisations', pp. 288–95, quoting H. A. Schatz.
54 T. H. Howell, 'Strategy and tactics of a geriatric unit', *The Hospital*, Vol. 64, No. 5, pp. 160–2. In the course of the article he quotes the work of J. B. Miner, *The management of ineffective performance* (McGraw-Hill, 1963).
55 L. Trotter and G. B. Adshead, op. cit., p. 425.
56 Ibid., p. 425.
57 D. Blaker and A. Hill, 'Practical developments in staff training', *The Hospital*, Vol. 67, No. 12, pp. 423–6.
58 M. W. Cuming, op. cit., p. 381.
59 Derek Williams, 'Diagnosing management training needs', *The Hospital*, Vol. 63, No. 3, pp. 100–2.
60 S. C. Haywood and F. W. Turner, 'A first-line management course', *Nursing Times*, Vol. 63, No. 31, pp. 1038–9.
61 D. Williams, op. cit., p. 102.
62 E. Jaques, 'Organisational structure and role relationships', *Nursing Times*, Vol. 67, No. 5, p. 155.
63 H. A. Simon, *Administrative behavior* (The Free Press, 1965), pp. 102–3.
64 Ibid., p. 103.

CHAPTER 18

1 Leader, *Nursing Times*, Vol. 68, No. 37 (1972), p. 1143.
2 'Money and management', *The Hospital*, Vol. 64, No. 8, p. 279.
3 B. Robb, *Sans everything: a case to answer* (Association for the Elderly in Government Institutions, 1967).
4 Report of the Committee of Inquiry into allegations of ill-treatment of patients and other irregularities at the Ely Hospital, Cardiff, Cmnd. 3975 (HMSO, 1969).
5 *Report of the Farleigh Hospital Committee of Inquiry*, Cmnd. 4557 (HMSO, 1971).
6 *Report of the Committee of Inquiry into the Whittingham Hospital* (HMSO, 1972).

7 National Health Service, *Annual Reports of the Hospital Advisory Service, 1970 and 1971* (HMSO).

8 National Health Service, *Annual Report of the Hospital Advisory Service*, 1971 (HMSO), paras 40 and 41.

9 E. Goffman, *Asylums* (Penguin, 1968), p. 302.

10 Ibid., p. 302.

11 See, for example, *Human relations in obstetrics* (HMSO, 1961). Ann Cartwright, *Human relations and hospital care* (Routledge 1964), chapter XIV. S. C. Haywood *et al.*, 'The patient's view of the hospital', *The Hospital*, Vol. 57, p. 644.

12 V. Carstairs, *Channels of communication*, Scottish Health Service Studies, No. 11 (1970), p. 29.

13 P.E.P., *Family needs and the social services* (Allen & Unwin, 1961), particularly pp. 31–40.

14 S. C. Haywood *et al.*, op. cit.

15 V. Carstairs, op. cit., p. 26.

16 A. Cartwright, op. cit., p. 203.

17 J. R. Ellis, 'Community medicine', *The Hospital*, Vol. 64, No. 6, pp. 194–9.

18 Ibid.

19 V. Carstairs, op. cit., p. 26.

20 E. Goffman, op. cit., pp. 281–336.

21 There are some conditions and aspects of medical care where this may not be so. For example, Routh reports on the constant negotiations between practitioner and patient on the controls on behaviour which were thought necessary for a therapeutic regime (Rose, Arnold (eds.), *Human behaviour and social processes* (Routledge & Kegan Paul, 1962)). This may be so too on the question of diets. Yet for most conditions the doctor's prescription is accepted; where this involves surgical procedures or a course of drugs there is no doubt that they are in the interests of patients. Hence there is no *major* clash of interests in treatment.

22 H. A. Simon, *Administrative behavior* (The Free Press, 1965), p. 16.

23 Ibid., p. 110.

25 Ibid., p. 111.

25 Ibid., p. 133.

26 *Report of the Committee of Inquiry into the Whittingham Hospital*, op. cit., p. 5.

27 A. Cartwright, S. C. Haywood *et al.*, op. cit.

28 V. Carstairs, op. cit., p. 26.

29 R. G. S. Brown *et al.*, op. cit., pp. 21 and 34.

30 Ibid.

31 Ibid., p. 34.

32 V. Carstairs, op. cit., p. 26.

33 Ibid., p. 26.

34 A. Cartwright, op. cit., pp. 192–4.

35 R. L. Coser, 'A home away from home' in *Sociological studies of health and sickness* (McGraw-Hill, 1960), pp. 154–72.

CHAPTER 19

1 E. Goffman, *Asylums* (Penguin, 1968), pp. 14–20, A. Cartwright, *Human relations and hospital care* (Routledge, 1964), Chapter 11, *passim.*

2 C. M. Taylor, *From person to patient: problems and progress in medical care* (O.U.P. for Nuffield Provincial Hospitals Trust, 1972), pp. 93–112.
3 Ibid., p. 107.
4 Ibid., p. 107.
5 Ibid., p. 108.
6 T. H. Howell, 'Strategy and tactics of a geriatric unit', *The Hospital*, Vol. 64, No. 5, p. 160.
7 H. T. Phillips and M. C. Larkin, *Hospitals*, Vol. 46 (16 February 1972), p. 55.
8 C. J. F. Williams, 'A patient's point of view', *The Hospital*, Vol. 64, No. 9, p. 308.
9 Ibid., p. 309.
10 Ibid., p. 308.
11 *Human Relations*, Vol. 13, No. 2 (1960), p. 113.
12 R. Klein and J. Ashley, 'Old age health', *New Society*, No. 484.
13 D. F. Phillips, 'The hospital and its dying patient', *Hospitals*, Vol. 46 (16 February 1972), p. 75. Report of a conference.
14 See D. F. Phillips, ibid. for summary of this argument. The book quoted is *Time for Dying* (Aldine Publishing Co., 1968).
15 Ibid., p. 75.
16 Ibid., p. 75.
17 R. A. Strank, 'Caring for the sick and dying', *Nursing Times*, Vol. 68, No. 6.
18 J. Cheadle, 'The rejected patient', *Nursing Times*, Vol. 67, No. 3, pp. 81–4.
19 Ibid., p. 84.
20 Ibid., p. 81. M. Y. Ekdowi, 'The difficult patient', *British Journal of Psychiatry*, Vol. 113, pp. 547–52.
21 Report of the Committee of inquiry into allegations of ill treatment of patients and other irregularities at the Ely Hospital, Cardiff, Cmnd. 3975 (HMSO, 1969).
22 Report of the committee of inquiry into the Whittingham Hospital (HMSO, 1972), para. 50.
23 Mrs J. Robinson. Letters to the Editor, *The Guardian*, February 2, 1973.
24 For a description and assessment of these tribunals read K. Bell *Tribunals in the Social Services* (Routledge, 1969), chapter 5.
25 White Paper on National Health Service Reorganisation, Cmnd. 5055 (HMSO, 1972), p. 55.
26 G. L. Cohen, *What's wrong with hospitals?* (Penguin, 1964), p. 111.
27 C. Kirk, 'Management and community participation', *Lancet*, Vol. 1, No. 7758 (1972), pp. 1006–7.
28 C. Kirk, ibid.
29 Ministry of Health, Central Health Services Council, *Human relations in obstetrics* (HMSO, 1961).
30 Ministry of Health, Central Health Services Council, *The pattern of the inpatient's day* (HMSO, 1961).

CHAPTER 20

1 The Annual Report of the Chief Medical Officer of the Department of Health and Social Security for the year 1970, *On the state of public health* (HMSO, 1971), p. 15.

Index

204